Praise for *Healing Yo*

"If you're the parent of a special needs child, ... find an empowering and refreshing way of viewing your child's condition. The information presented here will help you to understand what is happening, to get to the root cause of the problem and give you a roadmap for helping your child to heal. Recent studies are finding that our brains have a much greater ability to heal than is generally appreciated. In this book you will find a scientific, practical and well-researched method for assisting that healing process. During the years I consulted with families at Family Hope Center, I saw hundreds of children who surprised me with the progress they made on this program, well beyond anything I'd seen or been taught to expect in my pediatric training. If I were a child with a brain injury, I would be hoping that my parents would find this book and follow its recommendations."

—Linda Baker, MD, CCH, Portland, OR

"It is thrilling to see the decades of dedication spearheaded by Matthew and Carol Newell and their diverse team at the Family Hope Center encapsulated in this book. In it, their philosophy, approach, and results in overcoming neurological injuries—even the most severe cases—are made accessible to professionals and families alike. Yet beyond their extensive experience in the recovery of neurologically injured children, their work demonstrates exciting potential in the enhancement of well-being and achievement in youngsters of 'normal' families. I can attest to the brilliant results this program can elicit through its solid and well documented multidisciplinary agenda in nurturing families who deal with the enormous challenges of raising an injured child, and the benefits that spill over to siblings and parents. In the fullest sense of the word, the Family Hope program can 'raise' an individual to her fullest potential. This book provides a broad picture of previously unsuspected possibilities in neurological recovery and effective parenting."

—Nancy Werner, MD

"This book is so rich in enlightenment and knowledge of how parents or other close relatives can bring hope and development to children and adults suffering from neurological disorders."

—Mira Helena Bergkvist, MD, Sonderborg, Denmark

"As a medical professional, I've heard countless lectures in neurology and read numerous textbooks for courses. As a parent, I've had conversations with neurologists and neurosurgeons from the best hospitals this area has to offer. None of them can explain the brain like Matthew Newell does. He understands the brain and can easily describe any area of it and how it relates to function. More importantly, he understands it will be enough to teach you what you can do to make an impact on that particular area. The information I've learned from him has changed how I think, how I treat my patients, and how I raise my children. His book will be a game changer for those who take the time to read it and let it change how they think!"

—Dr. Stephanie Ale, DPT, Certified MDT, CSCS, Woodstown, NJ

"This is essential reading for anyone who works with someone with any type of brain injury, therapists and parents alike. Matthew Newell brings focus to the basic and most important aspect of rehabilitation, how to reach the central nervous system. His knowledge and approach bring hope to parents, injured and other family members. Parents will understand how to help their children and therapists will have the tools to work in a logical and methodical way to reach the potential in every individual they meet. This book should be a staple in every university level education that teaches about brain injuries in both children and adults."

**—Dr. Jörgen Sandell, PhD, Clinical Medicine,
MSc PT, DC, Stockholm, Sweden**

"I had the pleasure of meeting Matthew Newell when he attended one of my classes. Since then, I have had the opportunity to spend time learning from him and his exceptional staff. During my visits with Matthew, I have found him to be not only extremely gifted, but also incredibly focused and determined to find better answers for his clients. In the work he and his staff do with children who have brain injuries, he has found that educating parents and caregivers has been an integral component to the success of the program. With this book, Mathew can now share the wealth of knowledge he has accumulated over the years working with countless numbers of children with a wider audience and succeed in his mission to educate others beyond his program. I, for one, am grateful that Mathew has decided to offer us all his insight and experience by writing this book, and I know it will be an incredibly helpful resource for everyone who works with this special group of children."

**—Dr. Kerry D'Ambrogio DOM, AP, PT, DO-MTP, AdvCBI,
AdvCBP, SrCBI, senior practitioner and instructor for BodyTalk**

Praise for the Work of Matthew Newell & Carol Newell

"After suffering a stroke and severe meningitis, my 4-year-old son was left with right sided motor impairment, difficulty with short and long-term memory, spatial disorientation and sensory processing issues. As many parents who suffer the trauma of having a brain-injured child, we could see his heart and soul were still bursting with abundant life and beauty. As a physician, I was very familiar with the conventional treatment plan of PT and OT laid forth by his brilliant team of doctors at Boston Children's Hospital. I was struck by how these therapies addressed the symptoms (muscle weakness) rather than the root of the problem (a hurt brain). It made much more sense to me that we should be working on creating new neurological pathways rather than trying to fix the manifestation broken ones to work. The 3-day seminar led by the Newells and their team was a crash course in neurodevelopment which dovetailed beautifully with recent data around the science of neuroplasticity. They use detailed anatomical and developmental neural network maps in the brain to evaluate where along the timeline of brain development your child suffered injury, causing a dysfunctional pathway for that particular network resulting in downstream consequences. They design a personalized plan for each child based upon the particular sequence of neural dysfunctions and help strengthen the network from the origin of the dysfunction rather than fixing the symptom that is revealing itself. It is a complete multi-modal brain health approach: optimizing nutrition and fuel for neuro-regeneration, using physiology of breathwork to enhance oxygenation of brain tissue, incorporating body and energy work to repattern pathways, creating a unique sensory stimulation program, and returning to basic motor and reflex pathways such as crawling to develop a strong foundation for the most effective brain development. As parents, we are not just shown an action plan which is extremely empowering, but we are given hope, support and community. We saw significant gains after working on the program with our son for 6 months. Both his neurologist and neurosurgeon have been blown away by his progress. The program helps your child adapt and become more resilient, not just get 'band aid solutions' that don't promote his or her potentiality and evolution. Now I have applied aspects that I've learned from the program with my other children, myself and even my patients. I am excited to use the book as a resource in my office and share it with my community."

—Liz Strawbridge, MD, Maine Integrative Healing

"When I had my son, I felt many of the things that parents who learn that their child has neuro-development issues do: fear, a sense of loss, and more fear. If I knew what I know now, fear wouldn't even be in my vocabulary. We had been lucky enough to be directed to the Family Hope Center when my son was an infant. With a diagnosis of Down syndrome and a very nasty bout of a rare seizure type, my son has gone beyond 'thriving.' He is remarkable. He talks, walks, jokes, loves, reads and laughs like the master of his world that he is. We continue to expand his brain by use and the principles of the neuro-development program taught to us by the Newells and the specialists at Family Hope Center. There are no limits to what my son can achieve. I credit the sound principles, based in science and core neurology, and his team for helping him get there."

—**Madhavi Gupta Dyen, MD, Board Certified Neurologist, Upland, PA**

"I came to the Family Hope Center conference as an exhausted parent, a frustrated wife, a disillusioned academic and a resistant medical not-so-professional. I did not believe that 3 days of talking about what I presumed to be neuro-pseudo-science would change my outlook forever. I came heavily armed and guarded with a career of preconceived ideas, arguments, opinions and training about neuro-development. And I was gently persuaded to pack my weapons away without giving up the science. The Family Hope Center has the heart of the Healer that I have always longed to cultivate more fully—one who promotes ability and does not stop at disability. The Center focuses on ease, not disease; on full function, not dysfunction, on treats and not just treatment, on joy and not on sadness. I left the conference feeling contagiously overjoyed at how attainable and do-able the steps to healing can be. Complexity was exchanged for plain and simple truths, demonstrations, testimonies and results. Yet a sense of awe was maintained at how intricately the brain was designed. Simple ways to experience the magnificent. It was like being given a road map with milestones and beacons to follow through steep mountain paths. The Family Hope Center team has trodden and carved out these paths over years of research, experience and training. Their pioneering walk has made the path now possible for everyday parents to walk—everyday in their own shoes, in their own homes. And the paths bring thousands to new places and heights and viewpoints. As I sat in the conference, like being on a mountain top—my eyes were gently opened to realise how God has given us all we need for healing—the air we breathe, the water, the food, the ground under our feet and the love for our children, and it took my breath away. I will never be the same. And I am ever grateful that the Family Hope Center took me to the precipice; where I did not want to be challenged and with a safe guardrail of evidence and science opened my eyes to look over the edge at new frontiers of hope."

—**Dr. Shirley-Anne Jourdan, MD, GP, Pretoria, South Africa**

"Best thing to happen to our child and our family. I'm indebted to you for the rest of my life. My motherhood has been restored."

—**Lisa Keller, Ed.D., Associate Professor of Educational Policy, Research & Administration, UMass Amherst**

A Proven

Approach to Helping

Your Child Thrive

HEALING YOUR CHILD'S BRAIN

MATTHEW & CAROL NEWELL

BENBELLA

BenBella Books, Inc.

Dallas, TX

BENBELLA

BenBella Books, Inc.
10440 N. Central Expressway
Suite 800
Dallas, TX 75231
www.benbellabooks.com
Send feedback to feedback@benbellabooks.com

BenBella is a federally registered trademark.

Printed in the United States of America
10 9 8 7 6 5 4 3 2 1

Library of Congress Control Number: 2020946078
ISBN 9781950665433 (trade paper)
ISBN 9781950665587 (ebook)

Editing by Greg Brown
Copyediting by Scott Calamar
Proofreading by Sarah Vostok
   and Michael Fedison
Indexing by WordCo Indexing Services, Inc.
Text design and composition by Katie Hollister

Cover design by Sarah Avinger
Cover image © Shutterstock /
   LizavetaS
Printed by Lake Book Manufacturing

Distributed to the trade by Two Rivers Distribution, an Ingram brand
www.tworiversdistribution.com

Special discounts for bulk sales are available.
Please contact bulkorders@benbellabooks.com.

This book is dedicated to all parents and professionals who with love, tireless conviction, and hope believe that the brain can grow, children can develop beyond the labels, and families can heal.

CONTENTS

FOREWORD

by Dr. George Goodwin

As an internal medicine physician with more than twenty years of experience, I carried a high degree of skepticism toward alternative treatment systems that had not already been clinically proven. I received my doctor of medicine from the Uniformed Services University of the Health Sciences in Bethesda, Maryland. I am board certified in internal medicine. I had the privilege to serve for over twenty-five years in the army. During my career, I deployed twice, serving our soldiers in both Iraq and Afghanistan. I also was the chief medical officer for a military medical facility at Fort Eustis, Virginia. I culminated my career as a colonel in the Pentagon overseeing the disability program for our wounded warriors and directing all the medical standards for readiness in the army. All this experience was within what would be considered traditional medicine.

For my wife, Renee, and I, our journey began with a son who had developmental delays and social challenges in a spectrum disorder. We noted within the first couple of years that although our son was developing physically, he had severe difficulty interacting with others in normal social environments (preschool, church, and other social gatherings). We had our son evaluated several times. We were encouraged by both his teachers and conventional medical providers to put him on medication for ADHD, but never elected to do so. Instead, we were looking for alternatives to help him succeed. Therefore, when one of my colleagues at the Pentagon informed me of the work that Matthew and Carol were doing with their three children, I was cautiously intrigued. He shared the impacts that they were seeing in their children's progress, which was a personal perspective that I could see firsthand.

Renee and I chose to go to a three-day parent training conference to research the actual methodology being implemented at the Family Hope Center. Employing a very holistic approach, Matthew and Carol demonstrated the observable impacts they have seen over nearly forty years of clinical experience. During our time there, I studied all the material that was provided and researched as much medical literature as I could obtain on neuroplasticity and brain healing. Although I still did not fully understand all the underlying physiology of the healing that they were observing, Renee and I decided to partner with Matthew and Carol and the team at the Family Hope Center to see what impact it would have with our son and family because I was convinced that sufficient evidence existed in literature and in the early research that Matthew and Carol were completing.

We did have to make some changes in our life to integrate the holistic approach to obtain improvement for our son. The biggest changes were in our schedule (time management and calendar planning) and our diet. The whole family made some adjustments. However, the results were unquestionable. Our son's improvements in his physical abilities, social interactions, and application of cognitive learning were immense. I was unsure how my son would be able to survive in the world with the deficits we were seeing, but now we are confident that he will be able not only to survive but to thrive in the world around him.

As the fields of neurocognitive research, neural development, and brain healing continue to develop, it is exciting to see pioneers that continue to partner with families and to see clinical impacts in the lives of young men and women. Both as a physician and a father, I am thrilled to witness this work being published. It is imperative these perspectives on healing be shared. This book will begin to provide insights into the application of the principles that Renee and I have used to see the improvements in our home. These clinically proven results based on this fresh approach will positively impact more families, providing hope!

George Goodwin, MD
Internal medicine physician at Fort Belvoir Community Hospital, US Army colonel, and former Director of Disability Evaluations at the Office of the Surgeon General

INTRODUCTION

Shifting the Special-Needs Landscape

Autism. ADD/ADHD. OCD. Behavior-related disorders. Learning difficulties. Delayed and disorganized language. Genetic-based neurodevelopmental delay. Dyslexia. Epilepsy. Cerebral palsy. Down syndrome. Traumatic brain injury.

Think about the last night you really had a good night's sleep. From the moment you had the sinking feeling in your stomach that your child was struggling, to the moment when your child was diagnosed with one of these special-needs-related conditions, sleep has likely been scarce.

Sleep is difficult—perhaps even impossible—when you know that your child in the room next to you is not thriving the way they should. You toss and turn with worry and dread because you are concerned yet confused by what to do.

Perhaps you've already consulted with an array of doctors, specialists, therapists, and support groups, tried this and that, and now feel overwhelmed, ignored, misunderstood, marginalized, or disappointed by your efforts and by the outcome. You know that somehow, somewhere, you must find a way to help your child.

Well, we're here to show you that way—a way that has worked successfully for thousands of children. We're here to guide and support you and your family.

SYMPTOMS ARE NOT THE CAUSE

Over the last decade, you may have noticed or read about a substantial rise in the number and variety of neurological issues being discovered and diagnosed in our children, as well as an increase in reading, learning, and behavioral problems. Along with this trend, there's been an increase in the use of medication to manage *symptoms*. Symptoms merely indicate that a condition exists, and treating symptoms does not, and never will, foster healing. In fact, it does the opposite. For the healing process to begin, you must first identify and examine the *source* of the injury manifesting the symptoms. Very often, that brings us back to the brain.

The goal of *Healing Your Child's Brain* is to change the way you look at your child and their potential. We'll explore what is happening in the "hard drive" of the brain and how it is affecting your child's neurology. We'll explain how, when you stimulate specific areas of the brain, you will witness firsthand how those dreaded symptoms gradually disappear. Once you are on the real path—the path to wellness—you will see your child develop.

You'll discover what you can do to understand, support, improve, and help to heal your child, wherever they are on the continuum of neurological organization.

THIRTY-EIGHT YEARS AND MORE THAN TWENTY THOUSAND FAMILIES

Over the last thirty-eight years, we've taught and helped nearly twenty thousand families whose children have ranged in ability from very well organized to children who were blind, deaf, insensate, paralyzed, or so hurt that they required a tracheotomy to breathe and a feeding tube to be nourished.

We've seen children with every diagnosis imaginable at our office in Pennsylvania and across six continents. We can say with certainty that the vast majority of even seemingly "well" children have their share of neurological "bumps and bruises."

Few children achieve neurological advancement without significant support or intervention by their parents and healthcare professionals. So even if your sole intention is to find a new way to help your most vulnerable child, the odds are that every child in your family will benefit from what you learn here.

Our approach is bottom-up, inside out, and scientific based. We have documented results to back up our work. In fact, our program's success rate is sometimes nearly triple the national average, based on the WeeFIM assessment. (The WeeFIM is the most widely used system in the world for documenting the severity of child patient disabilities and rehabilitation outcomes. You can learn more about this at www.familyhopecenter.com/results.htm.)

Above all, we are parents, too. We have sat where you are now sitting and have dedicated our careers and our lives to helping and empowering parents to learn about the brain and gain the confidence and skills necessary to proactively engage with their child with special needs in a neuro-sequential manner.

OUR STORY

Our journey began as students, working in a university clinic (Matthew, in the US) and as an NNEB (diploma in childcare and education—Carol, in her native England). As young adults, we both trained under some of the most innovative practitioners in the field of brain development. We studied and received certifications in child brain development, and later in craniosacral and myofascial release therapy, infant parent mental health, and many other progressive therapies. We ran programs around the world for neurologically impaired children and teens. All these experiences and efforts eventually led us to establish the Family Hope Center in Norristown, Pennsylvania, in 2002, where we evaluate the neurology of children, and teach, guide, and support parents to implement comprehensive, individualized programs we create for each child we treat, fostering brain function and development.

On a personal note, we even met, married, and started our family while working with children. Our training and expertise were put to the test, however, when two of our children faced complex developmental difficulties.

Our son, Ben, met his developmental milestones in a typical manner. He is now a well-rounded adult who is working with us to establish a flagship school that will provide a comprehensive educational program for children with neurodevelopmental disabilities.

Our daughter Shayna started life as a healthy baby. At the age of three months, she had an adverse reaction and high fever in response to a DPT vaccination. While this correlation might have been a tragic coincidence or an anomaly, given the scientifically disproved concern regarding vaccines, we nevertheless witnessed her abrupt changes firsthand.

She developed strabismus, became hemiplegic (incapable of using one side of her body), and by the time she was school-aged, had developed severe learning problems. At the age of seven, she could still not read her name or identify the letters of the alphabet. It took nine years of daily, diligent effort to heal our daughter. She became an excellent violinist and competed at a high level in gymnastics. She now has a doctorate in occupational therapy and works at a hospital. She readily recalls the difficulties she had growing up, struggling to read and retain information. These tribulations challenged her confidence and self-esteem, which, in turn, made her fiercely committed to overcoming her limitations. Shayna remembers the intense programs we implemented to make her whole again. She lives in the present and appreciates the abilities she has now. She knows that her hard work—and ours—has paid off. As parents, we have the peace of knowing we were able to shepherd her through her injury and give her the best possible future.

We adopted our youngest daughter, Mary Taneisha, when she was five months old. She came to us with neurological challenges that made her cry for hours on end. It was heartbreaking and frustrating, but once we identified the root of her issues, we took steps to heal her as we did with her older sister. However, as she matured, additional intellectual and social challenges emerged, exacerbated by a sugar addiction. She was often impertinent, angry, and prone to harmful behaviors. Mary was stubborn and frequently railed against the neurotherapy she needed to do that would lead to her improvement. Of course, we loved her unconditionally and knew she needed our love, focus, and persistence in kind, so we found the strength to move through her conflicts and the chaos.

Over time, we balanced her brain chemistry and helped her to overcome her physiological and neurological difficulties and turned the corner. Her stubbornness transformed into strength. Now in her twenties, Mary has successfully graduated from college, where she was a championship athlete. She works as an EMT and as a fire department lieutenant. By neurologically organizing her brain, we were able to develop her potential and set her on a healthy path.

And we did it all as a family. We had to apply all the knowledge we gained throughout our careers and clinical work—and seeking solutions when we hit snags—to help our daughters overcome their respective challenges. The results didn't happen overnight—it took many years of learning, dedication, patience, tough love, and continued faith in the brain's ability to heal.

The result of this journey is that we now have *two* valuable perspectives to share with you—one as professionals in this field, and the other as parents with children possibly just like yours. We've been in your shoes. We know exactly how you feel, what you've been going through, and how resilient you can be. We empathize with and care about you and your child.

We also know what works.

That is why we are compelled to impart our knowledge and the neurological strategies necessary that get results so that you can become empowered and productive neuro-parents.

THE JOURNEY AHEAD

When you read and digest the pages that follow, you will quickly understand that making a shift in your perspective will take you from feeling hopeless to hopeful. By learning more about the brain, and how it can heal, you'll change your focus away from what your child can't do and toward what they *can* do.

You will learn:

- How to help your child based on his or her current capabilities rather than where they're supposed to be.
- About the seven key developmental areas that help you evaluate your child. These are critical to helping your child function successfully in daily life and are also the ones most medical professionals focus on at routine checkups.
- How to measure your child's current ability in each of these seven neurological pathways and how to support healthy, measurable growth in each of these areas. You'll receive guidance on what you can do to heal these dysfunctional or compromised pathways and get your child back on track.
- The areas of the brain responsible for each sensory, motor, and social function.
- How to create an ideal home environment for your child's neurological growth and gain insights into what causes brain injuries in the first place.

Throughout the book, we'll share stories about the children and families we've worked with and the obstacles they faced and overcame.

We will also present all these seemingly complicated ideas in a manner that respects your intelligence and your already limited time.

With few exceptions, every injury to the brain is capable of healing. No matter how mild or profound, we have rarely run across a brain injury that couldn't be improved or completely healed given enough time, the correct approach, and dedicated effort.

Since we contend that you know your child better than anyone else, as you become more aware of the source of your child's neurological injury and their current and potential capabilities, you'll be in the ultimate position to help them make progress.

We are going to help you take control of your child's destiny. You are the loving, determined parent who may currently be confused, but you are also relentless in your pursuit of creating a productive and satisfying life for your child. This book will begin to provide you with tools, knowledge, and guidance to make it all happen.

All the very best,
Matthew and Carol Newell

CHAPTER 1

SETTING THE FOUNDATION FOR HEALING

When a child is born, parents embark on a journey they've been planning for nine months. Their hearts are filled with love, joy, and optimism. They dream of a life for their child in which cherished milestones are reached: the first utterance of "mama" and "dada," their baby's first steps, first day at school, college graduation, engagement, and marriage. They dream of watching their child creating a life for themselves over the years.

For parents like you, the dream is eclipsed by a major complication at birth or by a series of increasingly worrisome moments in which you begin to sense that something seems "off." You may have witnessed a massive collapse of your child's neurological health or, over time, noticed small red flags in your child's growth such as delayed speech, lack of or difficult movement, slow motor-skills development, poor eye contact, and feeding or digestive issues. Developmental milestones that other children are reaching fail to occur. Concern, disappointment, and eventually, a feeling bordering on panic set in.

As we posed in the introduction, after you realized that your child had a problem, when was the last time you really had a good night's sleep?

We know what that's like—we've been there ourselves. When our two precious girls were young and hurt, we metaphorically slept with one eye open until we understood what was going on and what we could do to help.

When you witness, firsthand, your child's array of struggles, you begin a new, unpredictable, and existential journey—one without a clear road map—to seek and find concrete answers to the questions pounding in your head: *What is happening with my child? Is something wrong? What can I do?*

Examinations are made, tests are run, and in many cases, you come face-to-face with a doctor who delivers the unfathomable news of your child's diagnosis, and you realize that your child is now considered "special needs." At that moment, the dream feels shattered, your life derailed, and you have no clue how to get back on track or what the destination will be.

Perhaps you had a different scenario. Your child might have been developing on target, socializing well, excelling at school, and thriving. But in the blink of an eye, they went from healthy to profoundly injured due to a car crash, stroke, infection, physical assault, or a tragic accident. Suddenly, you were thrust into the chaos of coming to terms with everything that has transpired and wondering if your child's life—and your own—will ever be the same again. And that reckoning for you may be even harder to contend with because of the loss of "what was."

Maybe your circumstances fall somewhere in the middle. You have a child who can't read well or keep up at school, seems clumsy and uncoordinated, struggles to bond with or integrate into the family and community, has high anxiety levels and is prone to distorted behaviors that alienate them from other kids, and struggles against the classifying labels already being applied to them.

No matter what happened to your child, your life as a parent, which was already one of focus and purpose, has now transformed into a life of hyper-focus and hyper-purpose. You've likely been consumed by the need to read, research, and inquire continually about your child's diagnosis and the viable treatment options to help them. You may also be overwhelmed by the opinions of doctors, therapists, professionals, family members, literature, support groups, and other parents with whom you've networked. You may have tried one or two courses of action or tried everything, but nothing works. You may have lost hope altogether, having been told that there is little that can be done for your child and the best you can do is take them home, care for them, and love them.

Do any of these situations reflect your despair? If so, chances are you picked up this book because somehow you still have hope—a hope that is born of love and parenthood, a hope that defines you.

We want to provide you with a realistic, scientifically based path that can begin to dispel your fears, frustrations, and anguish. We encourage you to embrace this hope and to make a shift away from despair toward possibility. It all begins with a simple change of perspective: from *this* moment forward, the focus is not on what your child *cannot* do but what they *can* do.

Inside your hurt child is a precious and miraculous organ that is capable of manifesting growth and healing. The brain.

It is possible to change the structure of your child's brain—from the cells themselves to the connections between the cells. The process of the brain reorganizing and forming massive synaptic connections is called *neuroplasticity*. By harnessing the brain's ability to grow and change slowly and steadily over time, your child *can* make progress toward healing.

EMBRACING THE POSSIBLE

Okay, we know. You just read that last paragraph and you're thinking, *How can that be?* After all, up until now, you haven't been given any reason to imagine otherwise. You've reluctantly accepted the current and prevailing so-called "wisdom," a potentially limiting *belief system* based on information you've heard or read.

Here's a question for you: *What is the moon made of?*

As you were processing the answer to this question, did you, at any time, think "cheese"?

You now know that's not the correct answer, but at some point, in your childhood, you probably thought it was true because you heard it from a sibling or maybe even a parent or grandparent. When someone you know, love, and trust tells you something with emotion, you will take it at face value and believe it to be true. This can be called a myth. It's a widespread belief or tradition that has grown up around something or someone—an unfounded, false notion.

In fact, *any* widely held falsehood is a myth, and these myths influence our thoughts and intentions. Some myths are harmless, but others shape and drive our behavior by validating existing, yet false, ideas that prevent us from embracing new ones.

This type of powerfully learned event can become hardwired into our brains. Suddenly, if we're asked about the consistency of the moon, we subconsciously default to "cheese." In the case of our children with special needs, we can perpetuate unfounded myths.

Think of all the myths you've heard about your child's situation and the conclusions you've drawn in your mind that now shape your beliefs:

> "My child is autistic, and since there is no cure for autism, I can't help them."
> "If a child is six years old, their brain can no longer grow or change."
> "My child has cerebral palsy and will never walk."
> "Once you are blind for five months, you will always be blind."
> "Your child will never read above a third-grade level."
> "Seizures are bad and can kill you."
> "My child is stuck and will never get well."

Whatever you've been told and have come to believe about your child, their capabilities, and their future, and regardless of where that information came from, being forced into accepting these beliefs based on false information is counterproductive to progress. By reading this book, you're in the midst of challenging these beliefs. You're being open-minded to new concepts and possibilities.

Good for you.

Good for your family.

Good for your child.

The most significant misconception to immediately overcome is that your child cannot be healed. If that's what you've heard and come to believe, think again. The reality is—and it bears repeating—that if your child has sustained any neurologically based injury or impairment, there are ways to reorganize the brain so it can form new synaptic connections, which will ultimately help your child on the path toward healing.

In the chapters that follow, you'll become more knowledgeable about the brain in general, begin to understand more about your child's brain, and learn how to identify which parts of your child's brain are happy and which parts arc not so happy.

The function of appropriately targeted stimulation and output will determine the growth and structure of the brain. In other words, just like your muscles, *the brain grows by use.* The more we stimulate the brain, the more the brain will grow. This growth can happen even when your brain is ninety years old—it just needs consistent and energetic stimulation. We'll show you how to promote and sustain neurophysiological growth in your child. Most importantly, we'll help you see what is possible and how you can be in the driver's seat of your child's neurological life.

By focusing on *where* your child is developmentally—our starting point—and embracing what is scientifically possible, you will begin to feel more hopeful and upbeat. That change in your demeanor will not only serve to motivate you but also resonate with your child and your family. Together, you can defy the odds and dispel that erroneous myth that your child will "never . . ."

To prepare for the journey to what's possible, start by becoming more informed and, consequently, more empowered. You can achieve this by recognizing and embracing your pivotal role as a parent and by making a few fundamental shifts in your mindset and resolve. Some may come more easily than others, but if you take heed, maintain a sense of optimism, believe in yourself, and trust your innate wisdom, you will become more confident, more focused, and more effective in helping your child.

YOU ARE YOUR CHILD'S BEST ADVOCATE

Question: Who really knows your child best?

Answer: Without a shadow of uncertainty, *you do.*

This answer may seem obvious in principle, but when you are continually advocating for your child to doctors, therapists, counselors, and teachers, all of whom may confidently share their opinions about your child and what can and should be done for them, you might begin to doubt your ideas or instincts.

Don't.

From the moment your baby was born, *you* were the one who interacted with them every day. *You* fed, changed, played, and cuddled them, watching every movement, every mood, and every smile. *You* discovered their likes and dislikes of food, toys, people, and surroundings. *You* witnessed their first cry, first coo, and first laugh. The minute you sensed something was wrong or of concern, *you* were the first to notice and take action. And you're still the one who's there each morning when they wake up and you tuck them into bed each night when they go to sleep. You are the one providing unconditional consistent love and a steadfast commitment to seeking knowledge and exploring options and solutions. No one else knows or understands your child as well as you do.

Working with a trusted doctor, therapist, or another professional is necessary and essential, particularly during your child's formative years. These are people who should become part of your support team. But when it comes to basic maternal and paternal instincts and astute awareness, parents rule.

In fact, to confirm this stance, in 2016 we commissioned a research study in the United States with the Harris Poll, which found that nine in ten parents of a child diagnosed with special needs believe they or their spouse/partner have the best understanding of their child's development. Additionally, 90 percent of these parents also believe they or their spouse/partner have the most influence on their child's development. Furthermore, not only do these parents think they understand their children the most, but they also think they're in the best position to guide their children to positive futures.

Never underestimate your intelligence and innate understanding of your child. Trust your instincts. Trust your judgment. Take the lead in your child's well-being. You can always listen to and weigh the opinions of others, but, in the end, do what you know in your heart and your mind is best for your son or daughter.

You are the one who can and should take control of your child's journey. *You* are the one who can make things happen.

LETTING GO OF GUILT . . .

With few exceptions, parents who attend our parent training conferences or bring a child to our office come burdened with guilt.

"Maybe it was the wine I had while I was pregnant."
"I knew I should never have smoked in college."
"If only I hadn't taken Justin to the store with me the night of the car accident."

We also hear confessions of mothers about overconsuming chocolate, wine, sushi, or fast food; the impact of work, financial, or family stress; concerns over vaccinations; and a host of other reasons parents believe they may have contributed to or precipitated their child's diagnosis.

While it is true that some parents with severe drug or alcohol addictions are likely to compromise the neurological development and health of their baby, the fact is that the source of most brain injuries is not attributed to something a parent did or did not do. A baby that suffers a loss of oxygen or blood flow to the brain during a difficult birth is unexpected and tragic but not the fault of the mother. A child diagnosed with a genetic disorder is fated by a rare mutation or quirk of DNA. Epigenetic and environmental factors—mostly out of the control of either parent—can also hurt a healthy brain. None of these situations is directly the parents' fault. Nor is having a teenager who sustains trauma to the brain in a car crash. These are outcomes that no parent can necessarily anticipate or prevent.

It is natural to feel responsible not only for your children but also for their "challenges." Experiencing guilt and self-doubt is normal, but if it overwhelms your emotions, it can immobilize you. Instead of dwelling on guilt, remorse, and grief, it would be ideal to focus that energy on a realistic, proactive strategy to help your child.

Your child needs your thoughts and actions focused firmly on a positive path to wellness. You are not the problem—the problem is the problem. What you are is the *solution* to the problem.

Self-doubt, self-recrimination, guilt, and grief linger, and they will compete against your hope. These self-imposed judgments cloud your conscience and negatively influence your life every hour of every day. They are neither healthy for you nor beneficial for your child. If you want to heal your child, now is the time to let go of these paralyzing and false beliefs.

In our family, we did this by providing our daughters with a neurologically proactive strategy that we implemented with them daily. We executed a plan and did not have time to look backward. We focused on a forward view, rather than on a backward view. It required discipline to do this. It helped that we had a daily plan to support our children—and we saw progress. Progress brought hope. Hope brought strength. Strength kept our mojo vibrant.

The truth is: your son or daughter is a well child who became hurt. It's not your fault; it's not their fault; it's not God's fault. Though it may be difficult at first, you must try to shift those feelings away from heartbreak and darkness and toward hope and possibility. Pause for a moment, take a deep breath, and let go of that grief and guilt. You may have to do this more than a few times. If you can, though, everyone will win.

DISPELLING LIMITING BELIEFS

We've addressed what you may have come to believe about your child, but what about what you think and believe about yourself? What messages are you giving yourself?

"My child is out of control so I must be a bad parent."
"I'm not educated/trained/qualified enough to help my child."
"My doctor/therapist/mother thinks I'm too emotional."

Do any of the above ring true?

Many parents feel helpless or believe that they are unqualified to help their children. Others feel marginalized, relegated to sitting on the sidelines where they become discouraged and passive.

Sure, there are days when you're exhausted or hopeless or feel alone and unappreciated. You're only human. If you find yourself acquiescing to self-imposed, limiting beliefs or taking to heart a few potshots directed at you by others, take a moment to step back and reflect. Go for a walk, meditate, pray, hug your child—anything that will tune out the negative voices in your head. Remind yourself that you're a concerned and capable parent who's bound to have these moments. You're 100 percent justified in asking all the difficult questions and seeking solutions. Above all, never forget that you know and love your child best and, with the correct information and execution, can do great things for your child.

MAINTAINING A SENSE OF HOPE

As a parent of a struggling child, you might feel frustrated because you're facing a complicated situation that you don't fully understand but are driven to figure out. That drive is fueled by hope. So you set out to get some answers, thinking, *I'm going to learn how to help my child to walk.*

But sometimes those hopes get dashed. Has anyone ever said to you, "It's unrealistic to believe that your child can ever walk," or "Don't get your hopes up too much"?

We heard that about our kids, too.

You might find that others around you—even close family members who love you—discourage you from having hope because they are concerned that you'll be profoundly crushed or disappointed if things don't work out.

Don't buy into it.

Your hope for wellness is a blessing to your child and should not be undermined by whoever claims your intention is a "false hope."

Dr. Jill Bolte Taylor wrote a brilliant book called *My Stroke of Insight*, which is recommended reading. Dr. Taylor was a thirty-seven-year-old Harvard-educated brain scientist who suffered a massive stroke due to an exploding blood vessel on the left (and logical) side of her brain. Because of her medical training, she was miraculously able to recognize what was happening and seek help, and to observe the rapid deterioration of her mind as it rendered her unable to walk, talk, read, write, or recall any memory of her life.

In her book, she writes: "Recovery, however you define it, is not something you do alone. My recovery was completely influenced by everyone around me. I desperately needed people to treat me as though I would recover completely."

Dr. Taylor needed people to believe in her and to "out believe" her problem. The person most responsible for believing in her and her ability to heal was her seventy-year-old mother, who was her champion. It took eight years, but Dr. Taylor recovered. During that time, her mother never gave up hope.

She—along with thousands of other mothers and fathers we are privileged to know—maintained hope every day.

Never give up hope. Hope is good. Hope is an action word. Hope keeps you motivated. Your hope demonstrates to your child that you believe in him and his potential.

SEE YOURSELF THROUGH YOUR CHILD'S EYES

Sadly, many parents often see themselves through the eyes of professionals, and we know that is not a good idea. How many times have you entered a professional's office feeling confident and in control, asking questions or sharing articles you read, only to feel you're not being taken seriously? Sometimes you might even be told to calm down, stop being too intense, or to seek a support group. When your devotion and determination are unwavering, it can put unintended pressure on professionals, which they don't like. By the time you leave the office, you might feel minimized, insecure, or inadequate. You might even wind up acquiescing to the professional's point of view because of his education, credentials, and self-assurance. So when you view yourself through the eyes of professionals, you don't usually see yourself as capable.

We prefer and encourage a change in perspective—to see yourself through the eyes of your child. When your child now looks at you, all they think is how strong you are, how smart you are, how safe they feel with you. Perhaps, as a child, you were fortunate enough to feel the same way about your mom and dad.

Your child looks at you many times every day and, in their mind, they are asking themselves, *How am I doing so far?* If your eyes, facial expressions, voice, and touch reflect the judgment of a professional, your child will sense this insecurity. Despite the current circumstance, if you come across as a loving and hopeful mom or dad, your child will feel your optimism. How would you prefer to appear to your child?

When you continuously view yourself through the eyes of your child, you can maintain a competent and qualified attitude. And you *are* qualified. You can learn and do whatever it takes to help your child. It's a significant role to play but know that you are up for the task because you are determined, and this determination will give you the ability to help your child proactively.

Whenever possible, remember how your child sees and feels about you and your role in her life. Know that you have the right stuff.

REMEMBER TO BREATHE

Breathing is simple, right? So much so, you're not even aware you're doing it. But when your child is not doing well, you might find yourself holding your breath. We know—it's happened to us many times during the years of helping our daughters. It's difficult to breathe when you have so many things on your mind and responsibilities to keep up with: your child, the rest of your family, your home, and your work. It can overwhelm you. You're working so hard to get from point A to point B that it's easy to forget to breathe.

Whenever you have moments of stress or pressure that make you feel unsettled or uncertain, or if you notice that your breathing is erratic, pay attention. It's a sign you're not okay at that moment. Trying to manage everything day and night in a heroic manner is easier said than done, so try not to feel bad about being overwhelmed. Step back for one minute and take time to breathe.

Breathe in deeply for four seconds. Then breathe out slowly for four seconds. Repeat that process for sixty seconds. Pause for a moment and try it now. Feel the air in your lungs, in your brain, and down your spine. This simple task will help you regain your equilibrium.

PUT YOURSELF IN THE DRIVER'S SEAT

On the journey to your child's development, what position are you in right now?

Driver's seat? Passenger's seat? Back seat? Not even in the car?

If you answered anything other than "driver's seat," it's time to take the wheel and make a change.

Without realizing it, you may have been told or directed to relinquish control of your child's neurological path to others. You may be informed about what is happening, but depending on where you sit, you could be a passenger who is along for the ride with some input; or in the back seat where you view some of the journey; or else feel like you're not in the car at all and have little say or influence.

There are many reasons why you wind up as a passenger. You may be physically or emotionally depleted. You may not know what to do. Or you may know what to do but lack the confidence to do it. You may have repeatedly been told that others are more qualified and to yield to their guidance. You may be looking at all the credentials on the professionals' walls and feel timid about questioning their advice. While these reasons can contribute to not being in the driver's seat, we know all parents—including you—want to be at the wheel. What you need is a strong, reliable, and proven GPS—a neurological life coach who respects and validates your need to be holding the wheel.

As you begin to understand more about what is happening in your child's brain and learn about the appropriate tools and protocols that help that brain heal, you'll become more confident about taking the wheel. When you're in the driver's seat, you will consult your GPS and act accordingly. You can decide whether to take the highway or the scenic route; you can choose whether to travel at thirty, fifty, or seventy miles per hour. This is *your* family and *your* child.

When you're the driver, and in control, you have both intention and attention. You naturally pay more attention to the road ahead, knowing when to slow down or accelerate, knowing when it's time to take a break, and to appreciate the sights along the way. You also become more aware of the car and how it runs, fueling it with the right gasoline, and getting oil changes or tune-ups periodically to enhance its performance.

Our role is to show you a scientific and effective way to drive, using a method that has been "road tested" and proven successful for nearly forty years. That success is predicated on your being in that driver's seat. Once engaged—with joy and purpose—the days become very productive.

There's a quote by Thomas Jefferson that we share with every parent we work with and in every conference we give: "I know no safe depository of the ultimate powers of the society but the people themselves; and if we think them not enlightened enough to exercise their control with a wholesome discretion, the remedy is not to take it from them but to inform their discretion."

We have created our own version of this quote, which we wholeheartedly believe and want to share with you: "I know no safer place for families other than under the care of the mothers and fathers themselves. If we think them not enlightened enough to exercise wholesome discretion on behalf of their children, the remedy is not to take the responsibility from them and place it solely in the hands of professionals; the remedy is to inform their discretion by education."

We endeavor to inform and educate you so that you can create a plan and employ a solution that is reasonable and achievable. Our role—and the goal of this book—is to give you enough information so that you can take ownership of your child's healing, monitor the progress, and see the day ahead. Because, as William Drayton stated, "Change starts when you can see the next step."

Right now, you're probably spending your time putting out fires. It would be far better to be five minutes *ahead* of the fire rather than five minutes *after* the fire—that is a monumental ten-minute shift. Now you can begin healing instead of managing. Now you can become proactive rather than reactive.

With the right plan, hopefully, by the end of each day, you can breathe easier because you can see a way into the brain and now maybe—finally—get some sleep, too.

FAMILY SUCCESS STORY

Four years ago, my family was on the verge of breaking. We were scared, and unsure of our future. We were in desperate need of help with my siblings, and trying everything we could think of, but nothing seemed to work. I was only ten years old at the time, and I often found myself frightened of my little brother's outbursts and feeling neglected by my baby sister. I knew what autism was but didn't understand it. I wanted to help but didn't know how. But just when we thought we had tried everything, hope made its way to us. That summer, my mother attended the Family Hope Center's three-day parent conference and brought back the news that there was still a chance. She was ecstatic and could hardly contain her excitement. I can seldom remember a time when she was as thrilled as this. At first, I was wary of this new program. I was worried that it wouldn't work out, or that it would fail, as many others had, but after all this time, my expectations have been shattered by the results we have gained from these changes.

We started the diet almost right away and saw changes just as quickly. Liam, my younger brother, seemed happier, and more friendly. I began to feel less afraid of him and realized that it was the first time I saw the real him. And my sister, Aubree, gradually started to allow me to bond with her. It was like they had mental relief and could just be themselves. The diet isn't easy, and we now do home-cooked meals every day. I have even discovered new foods that I love. The extra work we've all put in has been worth it. We're healthier and happier now, and my siblings' personalities are at last revealing themselves to us.

The program itself is much more rigorous. We all have to do our share to make things work, and by the end of most days we feel exhausted, but it is worth it. My sister can speak and read, and my brother is showing more progress than we ever thought he would. I spend about an hour out of my day helping my mom with the program, and now know how to creep, crawl, do reflex bags, and other parts of the program with my siblings. My mom doesn't have to feel the weight of it all on her own. My dad and I are doing what we can in between work and school. Even my grandparents help! I know just how hard my family works and feel very appreciative of them. I've become confident in my ability to help, and I feel so proud of my younger siblings, and even feel a connection with them that used to be nearly nonexistent. I feel safer in my own home, and know that while things aren't perfect, my brother and sister are on their way to healing. Liam is no longer as aggressive as he once was, and instead is now very gentle and sweet. Aubree has stopped shutting me and everyone else out and has finally become like a true sister to me. I have gained far more empathy for those different from me because of this experience and program, and most importantly, my parents seem much happier and healthier than they have in a long time. Thanks to the Family Hope Center, we have once again become a family.

—Liam and Aubree's fourteen-year-old sister

NEURO-PARENTING POINTS

- It is possible to heal your child by healing their brain.
- As a parent, you know your child better than anyone else.
- Let go of guilt and grief.
- Release any negative beliefs you have about yourself.
- Never lose hope that your child will improve.
- See yourself through your child's eyes.
- Focus on your child's neurology.
- Become proactive, rather than reactive, about your child's well-being.
- Get in the driver's seat of your child's journey to healing.

CHAPTER 2

BEYOND LABELS: YOUR CHILD IS MORE THAN A DIAGNOSIS

Whenever we meet with parents, one of the first questions we ask is, "Can you tell me about your child?"

Take a moment to consider what *your* response would be. We're not talking about things like being sweet or funny. These are personality traits. Instead, think about your child developmentally. Does anything like the following come to mind?

"My child has seizures."
"My kid walks on his toes."
"My son's handwriting is illegible."
"My daughter's eye turns in."

If so, you're not alone. Sadly, most parents think of their child as a *collection of symptoms*.

When you observe that your child is falling behind other children and lacking development in a particular area, you can easily become so focused on the symptoms that you wind up using them to define and describe your child.

Perhaps you think about your child not by his symptoms, but as *a collection of behaviors.*

"My child has outbursts in public places."

"My son hits his brother."

"My daughter never listens to me."

"My son is rude and obnoxious to everyone."

Behavior changes and challenges can spring up in any child. But despite your best efforts to curtail them—whether you attempt to reason with her, give your child a time-out, ground her, or take away privileges—if the behavior problems remain unchanged or become exacerbated, this could be indicative of a more complex issue. And these behaviors now become the way in which you think of and define your child.

Is your child *a collection of disabilities*?

Many parents say:

"My son has a learning disability."

"My daughter is dyslexic."

"My child is physically disabled."

A disability is a catchall that can describe any deficiency or delay, regardless of severity. In fact, the United States government uses the term "disability" to characterize anyone with a condition for which specific rights are granted, such as special education or medical benefits. While these rights are essential and beneficial, society now identifies our vulnerable children by their disabilities—so much so that we now focus on disabilities rather than *abilities*.

What things *can* your child do? Can she read? Can she walk? Can she talk? Can you name five abilities your child has? Ten? When you think about it, you can probably find many abilities. But if you're fixated on the *can't*s, you may frequently overlook the *can*s. That's a point of view we encourage you to change. Why? Because all children have abilities, regardless of their extent. And when we focus on neurological abilities, we can help the child improve neurologically. More on this vital paradigm shift later.

Is your child *a collection of diseases or disorders*?

Some parents think of neurological disorganization or any diagnosis as a *disease*. The terms *disease* and *disorder* are often interchangeable, though a disease is more of an illness and a disorder is a disruption of a mental or physical function. If these are the lenses through which you see your child, you're apt to conclude:

"My child has cerebral palsy and cannot walk."

"My daughter is epileptic and is prone to seizures."

"My son is hyperactive and can't focus on schoolwork."

Many parents speak about how their children *got this* or *has that*. Once you put "got" or "has" in front of a disorder, that label can begin to define your child's identity. Your child can have a diagnosis, like autism, and you can honor that truth, without letting it define their identity or your thinking.

Is your child *a collection of syndromes*?

"My son has Down syndrome."

"My daughter has Rett syndrome."

"My child's vocal outbursts are due to Tourette syndrome."

Syndromes are merely collections of symptoms that characterize a condition that often has no known cause. They are usually named for the physician or scientist who discovered them. Some syndromes, such as Down syndrome, are genetic disorders. Regardless, they are yet another way in which children are defined.

Lastly, your child might be *a collection of guesses*. Have you ever taken your child to a specialist for whom you waited months for an appointment, and after an examination, you sat on the other side of their desk and got the distinct impression that what you heard was a guess? Some parents lament that their child baffled a specialist. Others have received uncertain or conflicting conclusions. We often hear something like this: "We went to the top doctor at hospital A and then to another specialist at hospital B. The first doctor said they think our child has PDD, and the other said they think our child has autism—now we're totally confused."

Maybe the specialist couldn't pinpoint the problem and presented a combination of diagnoses like "ADHD with the possibility of Asperger's syndrome."

The reality is your child is *none* of these things alone. These diagnoses, whether based on symptoms, behaviors, disabilities, diseases, disorders, syndromes, or guesses, are just labels. And *labels don't matter*—they are, by definition, a description and are not scientific.

BECOMING A NEURO-PARENT

What is a *neuro-parent*? It is a term we coined to get you thinking differently about your role as a parent to a child with special needs. It embodies the same qualities as a typical parent while encouraging you to look at your child through a new lens: that of your child's neurology. Even if you have other children at home who are developing and functioning as they should, the insight you gain from understanding how the brain develops will benefit *all* your children.

Later in the book, we'll explain everything you need to know about the brain and how to measure your child's current brain function—in a simplified manner—that will serve as the basis for evaluating his progress.

In the meantime, as you begin to focus on what is possible, let's explore other productive ways to look at your child and help him or her.

FOCUS ON THE NEUROLOGY, NOT THE SYMPTOMS

When you suspect that your child is different, and a doctor or therapist confirms your suspicion, the recommended treatment usually entails some aspects of therapy and managing the *symptoms*. If your child walks on his toes, he'll get ankle-foot orthotics (AFOs) on his feet. If her eyes turn in, she'll get a pair of glasses that forces the eyes to work in unison. If your son is hyperactive and unfocused at school, you'll be encouraged—sometimes even mandated—to administer a daily dose of medication to keep his behaviors in check. Many professionals are continually managing the symptoms because that is what they have been taught and trained to focus on. Managing symptoms does not address, and will never solve, the underlying neurological reasons for the disability, nor does it provide a remedy. It merely serves to make the symptoms less evident.

Our principle—and your role as a neuro-parent—is to focus on the neurology. We don't want to treat the symptoms; we want to look at the brain and how it functions. If the brain is happy, things happen one way; if it's unhappy, another. If you look at the output function of the child and the part of the brain it controls and something isn't right, that's where your time and attention should go.

Therefore, it is essential to understand the root of your child's symptoms, the degree of neurological organization, and to assess current abilities to determine where the child is in his development.

This is precisely why we use the term "brain injury." We choose to define this as the brain got "hurt" somewhere along the child's development, and that hurt is compromising their ability to progress and thrive. If we define that "injury" as some brain cells died and/or are underdeveloped, then we'd all be included in such a category. It's just not as apparent with some of us. We may all have a little disorganization, or a bit of incoordination. Perhaps we struggle to read quickly or read for pleasure, or are uncomfortable in noisy environments. But we've learned to maneuver around these "dings" and do well.

By gauging your child's growth, as compared to both the child and standard developmental milestones, you can measure how they're improving to the point of wellness.

Managing symptoms is, ultimately, not moving you toward healing from the inside out. With the proper therapeutic stimulation and opportunity, you can begin to heal your child's brain and promote neurological growth.

FOCUS ON THE DIAGNOSIS, NOT THE PROGNOSIS

When you sought the opinions and evaluations of professionals, you may have received a prognosis that your child will never walk, never graduate from high school, never have a family, never do this, or do that, and so on. That kind of stark feedback is not only fundamentally unscientific—because the brain can heal—but it is also professionally irresponsible.

It's not about the prognosis. A *prognosis* is a forecast on a future outcome. You are not psychic, and neither is anyone else. Even if you happen to be utterly tuned in to your child, you cannot predict the outcome or how long it will take Lindsey or Liam to get from point A to point B. What you can do is look at where your child is today and be proactive instead of reactive.

A proper neurological *diagnosis* is about identifying and explaining which areas of the brain are injured and *the extent* of the injury. Get a solid diagnosis. Assess and determine what is now happening in your child's brain and what areas need attention. Avoid setting limits or timetables on how poorly or well your child will progress. Whatever neurological plan you follow, measure its progress by using a valid measurement tool. This way, you will always know the pace of your child's development and adjust accordingly.

FOCUS ON NEUROLOGICAL, NOT CHRONOLOGICAL, GROWTH

For every parenting article or book you've read, and in every chat you've had with doctors or parents, you have probably focused on your child's age and what milestones she should be reaching. For example, walking by age one, talking couplets and phrases by age two, starting to read by age six, and so on. These all relate to *chronological* age.

However, a chronological developmental chart can't measure children with any special-needs diagnosis—their abilities must be measured neurologically. That means every child must be viewed according to the independent skills and abilities he or she consistently demonstrates. For children with special needs, chronological age and neurological age, by definition, are not in sync.

The ultimate objective is to have the neurological age catch up to the chronological age. That takes a scientific approach, a dedicated family, an innovative neurological team, and then the time and effort to consistently implement a tailored plan. Since every child is different, treatment must follow a program targeted to the specific areas of the brain that will actively promote neurological growth in that child.

Your child might be a ten-year-old chronologically, but his limbic brain may be functioning at the level of a five-year-old. If you focus on the neurological age (five) rather than his chronological age (ten), you will work more effectively toward building the appropriate neurological pathways so that these two "ages" can eventually converge. In other words, don't apply your energy toward where you *want* to be; direct your energy to where you *are now*, and then build toward where you want to be.

LABELS ARE FOR CANS, NOT FOR CHILDREN

In the medical community, the label applied when making a neurological diagnosis is merely shorthand—in one word or phrase—for classifying a group of related symptoms. This is understandable. It is more succinct to say "tomato soup" than it is to say "a mixture of pureed stewed tomatoes, milk, water, salt, spices, preservatives, and additives to give a creamy texture."

The therapeutic community devised labels as a handy but inaccurate and unscientific way to categorize groups of symptoms. These labels/descriptors also helped facilitate diagnostic coding, but they change almost every decade. When it comes to "brain injury," you would have been labeled as a "half-wit" as far back as the 1600s. During the twentieth century, the labels changed from "idiot" in the 1910s, to "moron" in the 1930s, to "retarded" in the 1970s. Obviously, these demeaning, offensive, and often misunderstood descriptors have been gradually replaced by terms more reflective of the social mores of the time. In fact, in 2010, the US Congress passed Rosa's Law, which changed the reference to "intellectually delayed." Clearly, labels have been around forever and will continue, but that doesn't make them right.

For some parents, labels often provide closure. Most concerned and anxious parents who know something is not right with their child, but don't know what the problem is, feel a sense of psychological closure—albeit temporary—once their child gets a diagnosis and a label. Sometimes, we want—we need—an answer, even if it confirms our worst fears. That label also puts us in "knowledge mode," whereby we can proceed to research the condition, read books, seek appropriate organizations, join a parent support group, and explore treatment options, because "now we know."

Labels can also be broad and inclusive of many symptoms and manifestations. For example, a diagnosis of *autism* denotes a child with speech delays, disorganization, hypersensitivity to sounds, tactility issues, and specific social anomalies. However, each of these individual symptoms is indicative of a separate neurological function with different areas of the brain being disorganized. Further, some children with autism speak while others do not. Some despise being touched, but others don't mind. Some children fixate and engage in stimming or other self-stimulatory behaviors, yet others do not. Some are high functioning, and some are not. The range of behaviors and functionality is so broad that the condition is now called *autism spectrum disorder* to accommodate the scope of characteristics exhibited.

But children and adults are not their labels, and labels do not define who they are or how they can heal. A package of symptoms doesn't identify the cause or location of the injury. Further, most medical professionals will differ slightly about how they perceive these packages of symptoms. That is why a child might be given different diagnoses from different professionals. This is confusing for parents.

We don't use labels because they are irrelevant and *not scientific*. They only serve to deter us from getting to the source of the neurological problem and formulating a solution.

FOCUS ON ABILITIES, NOT DISABILITIES

When a brain suffers a trauma or lack of oxygen, brain cells die. If a multitude of cells die in a specific part of the brain, the functions that are part of that particular area will be compromised, and a distinct set of symptoms result. Medical professionals have expended much time and energy toward classifying the various combinations of symptoms resulting from these types of brain injuries as well as an impressive list of names for these various combinations of symptoms. Regardless of these names, the diagnosis, or the condition, the result is that your child's brain is not functioning the same way it does in other children—and you want to understand why.

The error with labeling brain injuries is that each child—and each brain—is unique. A label only addresses the symptoms and not *where* the brain is injured or to what degree.

Instead of getting derailed by the label or the disability, we want to teach you how to identify and measure your child's unique abilities in each of seven critical neurological categories, which we'll cover in chapter five. As we touched upon earlier, the scientific reason we do not label children and treat their disabilities is that *the brain builds a successful hierarchical platform on foundational abilities, not on eliminating disabilities.*

Many professionals tell parents that there is no lasting neurological solution to ADHD (or to autism or Down syndrome or epilepsy, and so on). They recommend working toward eliminating the symptoms through medication, surgery, and other treatments—or doing nothing at all—and then moving the child through the school system.

Because of our science-based practice and decades of experience, we know your child has a full range of human potential in their grasp currently blocked in large part by a brain injury. The goal is to begin healing the whole child by starting from the inside and staying focused on healing parts of the brain rather than eliminating a multitude of symptoms.

When the focus is on disabilities, the tendency is to mask, suppress, and/or manage the symptoms so that the child appears functional. Treatment becomes symptom based and will invariably entail a combination of medication, strategies, devices, braces, or surgery. The assumption is that if you make the child *look* right, maybe they *will become* right. But we know none of that gets the child to a "yes"—it is merely a facade.

These types of approaches do not consider the brain's natural ability to form and reorganize synaptic connections. Rather than managing symptoms of brain injury, steps must be taken to heal it. Once you assess your child's abilities, you can work to develop and increase their progress toward normal progression. The focus is on building on what your child *can* do today. This is a neurological paradigm shift and an essential principle to understand.

You can begin the process by understanding more about the brain and how it works. Each part of the brain controls a specific set of functions. When you pinpoint where the injury lies in your child's brain, you can then target and develop that specific part of the brain. Our experience with both the concept of neuroplasticity and the positive results that have ensued demonstrates that the brain can grow based on a direct and consistent amount of stimulation. Over time, with a comprehensive, tailored plan implemented with consistency, the brain will begin developing, and the symptoms should begin to fade and be replaced with abilities.

FAMILY SUCCESS STORY

It was June 2006, and we were expecting our second daughter with great anticipation. All checkups during the pregnancy had been normal. In the early morning of June 25, I began labor unexpectedly and Isabella was born by C-section. Immediately, as soon as we received her, something hit us, and we felt our world fell apart.

When Isabella was born, she didn't cry, she didn't open her left eye, and it was noticeably smaller than the other. We didn't know what she had but we knew she was different. We felt and knew that something was wrong.

Later that week, during her first routine medical checkup, we were alerted by the doctors that Isabella couldn't see with her left eye and that she had a syndrome, probably Down syndrome. We just needed to put a "name" to it.

We were scared. Our greatest fear was that we didn't have the slightest idea of what we were facing. We began researching Down syndrome and committed ourselves to do whatever was within our reach for her. There were not many options of therapies for her in our city, just the conventional early stimulation activities they do for all the babies. No one expects a lot from children with Down syndrome; we were advised to take her to a daycare when she was two and then to school as any other kid.

Driven by our concerns, we consulted with another pediatrician who was recommended to us by our family doctor. This doctor was the first person to talk to us about a neurological developmental program in Philadelphia, assuring us that there were options for brain-injured kids.

That is how we had the fortune to meet Matthew and Carol at the Family Hope Center, when Isabella was two months old. We attended the parent teaching conference and began this journey. Time has proven to us that the effort has been worth it.

Attending the parent conference opened our eyes. We realized we had a lot to do for our daughter. We understood that the Down syndrome label was not the important thing; they taught us to understand our daughter and her abilities, and to help her move forward in her neurological development. One month later, we brought Isabella to the Family Hope Center for her individual appointment to develop her customized program. With their support, we did the program for seven years. We were taught how to organize her brain through movement, sensory stimulation, respiratory therapies, and nutrition, while strengthening the link among all our family members.

Thanks to this approach and guidance, we passed from days of uncertainty to a future of hope and optimism. In turn, Isabella became a positive, lovely, independent, and responsible girl who is always ready to help any person who needs it. Her language is surprising, and she is completely connected with the world that surrounds her. She was able to enter a regular school where she learned to read, write, add, subtract, and multiply at grade level, winning academic awards. She overcame many of the difficulties that children with Down syndrome have, leading a normal life. In fact, we usually forget she has Down syndrome. Other parents of children who were struggling in school looked at her progress and decided to attend the Family Hope Center, too, obtaining incredible results with their children.

God has always shown us a path with Isabella. She is our middle child and the center of our whole family. Thanks to the opportunity she had to organize her brain, we know she'll go far in life and beyond her label.

—*Daniela de Roux, Isabella's mom*

NEURO-PARENTING POINTS

- Many parents describe their child as a collection of symptoms, behaviors, disabilities, diseases or disorders, syndromes, or guesses. The reality is that your child is none of these.
- Your child should not be perceived as or defined by his or her diagnostic label, as it's not scientific.
- The brain matures by enhancing abilities, not managing disabilities.
- The symptoms and behaviors indicative of your child's diagnosis are all signs of a neurological impairment or brain injury that can be healed.
- Once you determine the injured area of the brain, you can create and implement a therapeutic strategy to develop and heal the affected area.

CHAPTER 3

MOVING FORWARD TOGETHER WITH MY CHILD

The question asked by nearly every parent of a child struggling or given a special-needs-related diagnosis is: "What happened to my child?"

That's a complicated question to answer because each child is different, and each situation is unique. While a professional can examine a child and make a diagnosis, there may be a myriad of factors influencing the cause of that diagnosis, some of which may be difficult to pinpoint. Many parents find living with this uncertainty frustrating. Many struggle with an unrelenting need to know. Hearing a diagnosis from a doctor brings some relief, but that often proves temporary as questions about what happened to the child—and why—still loom large.

HOW DOES A BRAIN BECOME INJURED?

Most diagnoses classified under the special-needs umbrella are likely due to an injury to the central nervous system. Impairment to the brain's function can occur before, during, or after birth.

Brain injuries don't spontaneously appear without cause. There are many ways in which a brain becomes injured, and the extent of the damage can range from mild to profound. Let's look at those that are most common.

GESTATIONAL CONDITIONS AND TOXINS

During the nine months between conception and birth, the health and well-being of a mother can have an impact on a growing fetus. The first trimester is a particularly critical time during which a baby's organs are forming. Smoking, consuming alcohol, and using many drugs cause known risk factors to a developing fetus. Fetal alcohol syndrome is particularly hazardous, leading to weak growth physically, physiologically, and intellectually, as well as to severe complications to the central nervous system.

Many over-the-counter medications, like aspirin, along with an array of prescription medications and various cancer drugs, are also known to be harmful. Exposure to certain illnesses, bacteria, and viruses—especially those for which a mother has not been vaccinated—can be passed to the womb and negatively impact a baby's development.

Conditions that are known to cause neurological damage include:

- Toxoplasmosis: This is a parasite acquired through consumption of undercooked meats, unwashed vegetables, or direct contact with cat feces.
- Rubella (German measles) and varicella (chicken pox): These are once-common childhood diseases that are now rare due to routine vaccinations.
- Sexually transmitted diseases (STDs): In particular, genital herpes, if active during the time of birth, can cause damage to the brain.

A mother can also pass along chemicals through the womb during pregnancy. Most of these toxins go unnoticed, but a simple urine analysis might reveal heavy metals in the mother's system, which can be dangerous to an unborn child. Undergoing dental procedures early in pregnancy, particularly the insertion or removal of mercury fillings, can also be detrimental to the fetus.

A mother who is obese or diabetic faces potential higher risks and should be monitored by a doctor. Some women develop preeclampsia, a dangerous, midterm pregnancy–related condition that is characterized by hypertension, protein in the urine, and fluid retention. In turn, this can affect the placenta and curtail the flow of oxygen and nutrients that are critical for fetal growth. This condition is severe and can cause damage to both the mother and baby, prompting the need for preterm birth and all the associated risk factors of prematurity.

Finally, there are physiological factors. Neural tube defects can develop in the early weeks of pregnancy during the formation of the spinal cord and brain, which can lead to conditions like spina bifida (an exposed spinal cord) or anencephaly, in which parts of the brain cease to develop. While some of these congenital disabilities can be traced to a deficiency of folic acid during gestation, there are other times when it is difficult to determine why the brain fails to develop fully.

BIRTH-RELATED COMPLICATIONS

The birth process, while biologically natural, can become complicated by factors that are not always foreseeable or preventable. For example, as a baby moves from the womb into the birth canal, the umbilical cord can wrap around its neck in a manner that constricts blood flow. Since a developing fetus receives its blood and oxygen through the mother's bloodstream and the umbilical cord, if the cord becomes tangled or compressed, there is potential for the fetus to become oxygen deprived for an extended period, resulting in brain-cell damage. This loss of oxygen is called *anoxia*. Anoxia is the number-one cause of brain injuries in children. It can occur in utero, during birth, or even after delivery.

Other brain-related injuries may ensue from a premature detachment of the placenta, the baby's head compressing against the pelvic bone during a difficult delivery, improper use of forceps or vacuums, and from some sexually transmitted diseases that are active at the time of birth.

TRAUMATIC BRAIN INJURY (TBI)

When the brain becomes injured due to an external force, it's classified as *traumatic brain injury* (*TBI*). Children are active by nature and enjoy playing with others, whether at the playground, schoolyard, or through organized sports. Getting hit in the head by a ball, or colliding with an object or another person, can lead to a head injury. Falls, in particular, are the leading cause of TBI. In fact, TBI is a common cause of disability and death in children and adolescents in the United States, with those from birth through age four being the most vulnerable.

Other traumas to the brain can occur through an automobile accident, drowning, choking, physical assault, or shaken baby syndrome.

ENVIRONMENTAL TOXINS

Even when a mother-to-be is judicious about her health, toxins in the immediate environment might affect a developing infant. Consider the Flint, Michigan, water crisis in which inadequate water treatment resulted in high levels of lead contaminating the water supply. More than one hundred thousand residents were exposed, including thousands of children whose health became severely compromised, especially in the brain and nervous system.

Toxic chemicals present in the air we breathe, the water we drink, and even in the food we eat can result in brain injuries. Most of the time, we're not aware that these toxins are present. Even if we take measures to minimize the risk by consuming organic food and filtered water, and using only natural cleaning and hygiene products, it's impossible to have total control over all potentially adverse environmental factors.

Exposure to heavy metals, particularly lead, is a leading source of brain injuries. Lead poisoning has resulted in brain injuries since the time of the Roman Empire. Efforts to eradicate lead from household products have been steady and successful. For example, lead house paint, which was common until the 1970s, has since been banned.

A study conducted by distinguished members of both the Harvard School of Public Health and Mount Sinai School of Medicine, and published by the *Lancet* Neurology in 2014, confirmed that there are close to a dozen chemicals that have been consistently linked to low IQ and compromised brain function. In addition to lead, these include mercury, PCBs, manganese, DDT, and fluoride. These toxins and others are present in fish, water, pesticides, cleaning solvents, flame retardants, gasoline, and some hair-care products and treatments used at beauty salons. The list of environmental toxins continues to grow, and prenatal exposure can have grave consequences for a developing baby as well as during early childhood.

ENVIRONMENTAL TOXINS CAN IMPACT FIVE GENERATIONS

If pregnant women are exposed to even low levels of lead, it can pass through the placenta and affect the developing brains of their unborn babies. Lead is known to have detrimental effects on the brain, causing impairment to learning and memory. Furthermore, in 2015, a research team at Indiana's Wayne State University discovered that high levels of lead in a mother's blood not only affects the fetal cells of her unborn children, but also the cells of her grandchildren. This is incredibly disturbing since most parents were totally unaware of how their exposure to lead predisposed their children—and grandchildren—to compromised health and neurological development.

In another study, previously undertaken by Washington State University, researchers concluded that environmental toxins caused ovarian disease across generations. Michael Skinner, founding director of the Center for Reproductive Biology at Washington State University's School of Biological Science, who was involved in the study, stated, "What your great-grandmother was exposed to when she was pregnant may promote ovarian disease in you, and you're going to pass it on to your grandchildren."

In a more recent study, Skinner focused on how embryos exposed to mercury passed on toxic effects to both their offspring and a third generation. Mercury, a neurotoxin known to cause brain injury, gets released into the environment through a variety of industrial-related sources and is carried by rain into our lakes and oceans. This is why pregnant women are advised to avoid eating many types of seafood, particularly raw fish and shellfish. This demonstrates, yet again, how the environment can become an insidious factor in both the biological and neurological development of our children.

GENETICS

Genetic causes of brain injury do exist. However, that in no way means they aren't healable. Down syndrome, one of the most common genetic conditions, is caused by the presence of a third copy of chromosome twenty-one. The extra chromosome compromises neurology, especially the respiratory system.

Most genetic brain disorders occur because of a gene mutation. While most are inherited, environmental factors can play a role. Genetic conditions known to impair brain function include:

- Leukodystrophy: A group of disorders that target the myelin sheath and can affect movement, speech, vision, and physical and mental development

- Phenylketonuria (PKU): The body's inability to process certain proteins
- Wilson's disease: A rare disorder in which the body cannot process copper
- Tay-Sachs: A metabolic disorder caused by a fatty buildup in the brain, prevalent mostly among Ashkenazi Jews, French Canadians, and Louisiana Cajuns. Although carriers of Tay-Sachs can be screened in advance of conception, it is usually impossible to screen for and prevent other conditions that may be caused by random genetic mutations.

Having a genetic-related condition, in our clinical experience, *doesn't* prevent the brain from healing. Through a customized neuro-sequential therapy program, a child with Down syndrome can make significant progress, as can those with other genetic conditions.

VIRUSES AND BACTERIA

In addition to infections that can be passed to a child by the mother during pregnancy, there are other viruses contracted during childhood that can attack and destroy brain cells. Fevers, while of concern to most parents of infants and small children, are a natural way for the body to fight off a virus or illness. They should be monitored and, in some cases, treated with over-the-counter medication like acetaminophen and ibuprofen. However, fevers that are brought on by heat exhaustion or heat stroke, in which body temperature reaches 105 degrees Fahrenheit or higher, are very serious and should be treated immediately; otherwise, injury to the brain will likely occur.

Bacterial meningitis is a serious condition caused by an inflammation of the membranes that line the brain and spinal cord. While some children contract and recover from meningitis without complications, others may experience an onset of vision and hearing issues, developmental delays, kidney failure, muscle problems, and seizures.

IMMUNIZATIONS: CAN THEY TRIGGER A BRAIN INJURY?

Immunizations are and continue to be a source of controversy. There is a continual debate about whether or not some cause brain injury, particularly as it relates to autism. Over the course of our careers, we have consulted with many parents who wholeheartedly assert that their kids were healthy until they were vaccinated, at which point they began exhibiting symptoms such as mild fevers, disorganization, listlessness, seizures, and emotional disconnection from the family. Is there a connection here? Or is it a coincidence?

We know that the overall benefits of immunizations outweigh the risks of contracting the diseases they prevent. We also know that although the chances are slim, every drug and vaccine on the market can cause side effects. Given that the average American child will be immunized to prevent the onset of about a dozen diseases, there will always be a small percentage of children who will have sensitivities, allergies, or other adverse reactions, and therefore contend with the aftereffects.

If you have observed your child experiencing an adverse side effect or illness after receiving a vaccination, you can report this to the Vaccine Adverse Event Reporting System (VAERS), established by the Centers for Disease Control and Prevention (CDC). Learn more at www.vaers.hhs.gov.

OTHER FACTORS

Sometimes, brain injuries occur from a combination of the factors mentioned above or even from seemingly rare and spontaneous conditions like a stroke. Brain tumors affect more than 4,600 children and adolescents each year. Poor nutrition and vitamin deficiencies in early childhood can also compromise neurological development.

If you have adopted a child from overseas or have little information about a child's family medical history or environment, there may be factors that have contributed to your child's neurological challenges. Articles published and studies conducted about adopted children from some orphanages confirm how the lack of nurturing, attention, and physical contact negatively impact the neurology of a child. This deprivation stunted the physical, neurological, and emotional development of these children. For many of these children, once caring families adopted them, they began to make progress.

Knowing more about what happened to your child may provide some clarity or closure or even alleviate a sense of guilt. If you intend to have more children, this understanding may make you more informed about any genetic predispositions to consider before undertaking another pregnancy. It can also serve as the first step to understanding more about the basis of your child's injury and how it is displayed.

IDENTIFYING NEUROLOGICAL CHALLENGES

Because we are parents, we are observing and making sure our children are on track in all the important ways. When we notice that our child is struggling, we will utilize all the available avenues possible to identify the root cause of issues we are seeing. Below are four common ways to verify our concerns.

IN FUNCTION

Brain injuries are *always* displayed in your child's function. You may notice that your child's eyes turn in toward their nose or point outward. Maybe they waddle when they walk, or stumble and fall often while running. Perhaps they tie their shoes without looking at them or by looking out of the side of one eye. Maybe your child doesn't speak well, has trouble pronouncing words, or coming up with the right words. They might put their hands over their ears when there's a loud noise or run screaming from the room. Or you might observe that your child bursts out laughing whenever their little sister starts to cry.

If you notice that your child moves, speaks, or behaves in ways that are underdeveloped or that deviate from the norm, these are indications that there is a neurological complication in the brain.

IN THE BIOCHEMISTRY OF THE BLOOD

Brain injuries are also seen in the blood. Certain chemicals in the blood have been identified as markers for specific types of brain injuries. One example is the level of essential fatty acids (EFAs). EFAs are vital for the development of the myelin sheaths around nerves and brain cells, as well as for hormone production. If these levels are too low or too high, they can affect the brain and nervous system.

Children exhibiting poor coordination or delayed motor skill development frequently lack EFAs. DHA (docosahexaenoic acid), which is an omega-3 fatty acid, is also essential for a healthy brain and brain function. In addition, it supports retinal development, which is critical to improved vision and eye function. The good news is that when we change the blood chemistry through appropriate nutrition and other forms of therapy, these injuries improve.

In recent years, researchers at Johns Hopkins University School of Medicine have discovered and continue to work on blood tests that can gauge the extent of a traumatic brain injury through measuring biomarkers and proteins in the blood. The results obtained will determine the severity of a concussion or TBI and facilitate the best course of treatment for positive outcomes.

Promising research at the University of Warwick in the United Kingdom is also leading to the development of biomarker-based blood tests for early detection of autism spectrum disorders.

IN A CT SCAN, MRI, OR EEG

CT scans, MRIs, and EEGs can show brain malformations and brain lesions that result from an injury. However, these diagnostic tests cannot provide the cause of an injury or whether there is damage to the brain cells.

Some scans of children's brains can appear normal even if these children are not functioning well. That's because these brain injuries are taking place at the cellular level that a scan cannot detect. So while scans may help in determining a traumatic brain injury, they may not prove effective in diagnosing other types of injuries or conditions. It is also important to realize that all these images are taken in real time and should *not* be used to determine a future prognosis.

We have seen a good number of children who, after following a neurological program for at least eighteen months, achieve significant, positive changes in the brain, which are confirmed by follow-up scans.

An example of this is a young boy who suffered a massive injury and needed a shunt. After the shunt was put in, this was a scan of his brain:

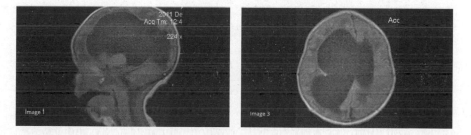

Thirty-seven months later, new images showed dramatic improvements.

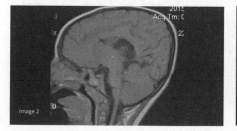
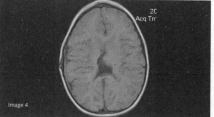

The boy's parents were following our recommendations for developing their child. These results serve to confirm that the brain grows by use.

IN THE OPERATING ROOM

Brain injuries can also be detected during surgery. Surgeons can look directly at lesions in the brain after a stroke or TBI. These injuries, which are large enough to be seen with the naked eye, are usually severe, making surgery vital.

THE MANIFESTATIONS OF NEUROLOGICAL INJURIES

Since we've established that, as parents, you know your child best and keep track of every developmental milestone reached, you are most likely to be the first to notice when something doesn't seem right or if there is a delay in your child's development.

When the brain is hurt or not working optimally, it can manifest the dysfunction through physical symptoms, such as:

- Lack of movement or poor coordination
- Disruptive social behaviors
- Intellectual challenges with reading, language skills, and comprehension
- Respiratory complications
- Seizure activity
- Metabolic issues
- Under- or oversensitivities in hearing, touch, taste, and smell

If you remain vigilant and recognize these signs, you can intervene promptly.

In subsequent chapters, we will discuss which areas of the brain are manifesting these symptoms or dysfunctions. For now, what follows are various symptoms your child may be displaying that warrant further attention.

POOR VISION

Many vision problems are neurological in origin.

Strabismus occurs when the eyes do not properly align. This condition can present itself as cross-eyed, a wandering eye, lazy eye, walleyes, or nonaligned eyes.

Lack of consistent ability for the eyes to track side to side and converge one's vision is a neurologically based disorder that creates difficulties in walking quickly and accurately on unpaved or uneven roads or grass in a yard, going up and down steps, reading or making eye contact, picking up objects, and playing sports. Lack of visual tracking and convergence can profoundly affect the child's ability to feel safe and secure within his environment.

Lack of depth perception occurs when the brain is unable to correctly connect and process the vision in each eye so that together the eyes can converge and thus create an image in three dimensions. Good depth perception is important because it can help to automatically assess distances between objects and how fast an object is approaching. Have you ever seen a child playing catch who, after intently tracking a ball, loses sight of it at the last second and the ball hits them in the head? Chalk this up to a lack of depth perception.

Neurologically, the eyes can drift randomly in multiple directions and cause major confusion for the child due to double vision and lack of depth perception. This double vision can also disturb the child's equilibrium and induce a feeling of nausea.

Nystagmus (also called "dancing eyes") is a condition that causes uncontrollable eye movement and it's a symptom of a brain injury. Since having nystagmus makes it challenging to sustain a steady gaze, it will also impair vision convergence.

COULD A CHANGE IN BEHAVIOR INDICATE A VISION PROBLEM?

Do you have a child who was doing well at school, but when he entered third grade, and the print in his books decreased in size, a problem suddenly emerged? You might have noticed that he was not keeping up with his work, developed some behavior problems, or started to hate school. If this happened to your child and you're feeling concerned, consider that this change could be due to a vision problem stemming from a neurological issue.

In most American schools, the print size in books, workbooks, and other materials reduces sharply somewhere around the third or fourth grade, just as the amount of homework begins to increase. We propose that many kids who develop behavior problems at school have, in actuality, reading problems caused by vision issues associated with neurological dysfunction within the central nervous system. When the problem is neurologically based, the use of corrective lenses or surgery puts a "Band-Aid" on the injury, managing—rather than identifying and resolving—the underlying cause.

The same situation occurs in the seventh grade when the volume of reading required increases dramatically—upward of fifty to one hundred pages of reading for homework each night. If you see a change in your child's ability to keep up with the material (regarding speed and comprehension), notice increasing agitation, and his or her grades beginning to decline, consider that this might be due to a vision issue stemming from a brain injury. As we mature, life becomes more complicated neurologically, and some children cannot keep up with the increased workload.

POOR OR SLOW READING

Reading ability develops more readily in some kids than in others—it is all about the brain. In addition to visual issues, some children have difficulty hearing the correct sounds of vowels and consonants, which will prevent them from recognizing whole words by sight or by reading phonetically. Difficulty in recognizing and processing words or in reading, writing, or spelling words is called dyslexia. Children with hemispheric dominance issues may also randomly reverse letters and numbers at times, making it incredibly frustrating to read.

POOR ATTENTION OR FOCUS

If you ask your child to do something, do you find you have to repeat the request numerous times before they comply? Or if you ask them to complete a simple task such as "Please go get your hat and jacket," do they return a few minutes later asking what it was they were supposed to get? Maybe they go for their jacket and hat but see a toy nearby that captures their attention and begin playing with that toy instead. This lack of focus and distractibility may be an ongoing issue in multiple scenarios.

POOR HEARING

Poor hearing covers several categories of symptoms. For example, there's the child who is hyposensitive to sound, meaning he has reduced sensitivity to or awareness of sounds. On the other side, a child who is hypersensitive cannot tolerate stark or loud noises—like a vacuum cleaner, restaurant hubbub, or people singing—when exposed to them. There is also the child who can't locate where a sound is coming from. If you call him from his left, he looks for and responds to the sound in the opposite direction, so he winds up confused—and so do you.

Another example of poor hearing is the *inability to perceive inflection* in the tone of another's voice. Perhaps Dad yells at Johnny to stop teasing his sister, and Johnny doesn't stop. Dad raises his voice even louder and says to Johnny, "Can't you tell I'm really serious about that? I told you to stop teasing your sister." The problem is that Johnny doesn't realize that Dad is serious because he cannot "interpret" the obvious inflection in Dad's voice. This child might also be unable to pick up subtleties like sarcasm or humor in vocal expressions.

When spoken to in a crowd or a public place, some children have difficulty filtering out background noises or other distracting sounds. They become anxious and exhausted, sometimes irritable, or may begin to cry. These responses can indicate a problem with how the brain processes sound.

POOR COORDINATION

Some school-age children may trip over their own feet, walk unsteadily, or frequently bump or run into other children. This type of poor coordination or clumsiness could be a sign of developmental coordination disorder (DCD). DCD will affect balance, fine motor skills, running, and jumping. Some children with DCD also have trouble holding objects, so this can cause problems with writing, drawing, and playing sports.

POOR SENSATION

Children who are undersensitive or overly sensitive to touch, pain, or temperature have *poor sensation*. Examples of this would be having a lack of or an adverse response to being hugged, or not laughing or crying when tickled. This lack of sensation may also be observed in the child who doesn't feel cold in the winter and goes outdoors without a coat or continues playing after sustaining an injury because he's not feeling pain.

It is common for kids with severe sensation issues to be misdiagnosed with a motor problem. If they can't feel their body, it becomes nearly impossible for them to express movement.

STUTTERING

Stuttering is a speech disorder due to neurological disorganization.

Most stuttering begins during the toddler and preschool years when children are developing high cortical dominance (genetically hardwired by parents) along with sophisticated language skills. Stuttering occurs through a lack of neurological dominance, i.e., left hand/eye/ear/foot versus right hand/eye/ear/foot. If the child cannot establish dominance or is overencouraged to use only their right hand, this can cause neurological confusion.

Language should come out of the dominant side of your brain, but in the case of a child who stutters, both hemispheres of the brain are firing language signals simultaneously. Stuttering is the result.

POOR LANGUAGE SKILLS

Poor language encompasses difficulties in verbal output, clarity, content, retrieval, or organization. You will notice this in the way a child expresses himself verbally. He may be unable to communicate thoughts in an organized manner, speak clearly, repeat phrases or omit keywords in a sentence, or have trouble learning words or using them correctly.

POOR CONCENTRATION

When kids have trouble focusing and keeping up at school, can't watch a movie or read a book all the way through, or have difficulty finishing any project or thought through to completion, this is due to poor concentration and focus.

POOR WRITING

Writing that is reversed, upside down, oversized, disorganized, or shifted can indicate a brain injury. Many children can read well but exhibit poor writing when printing words on paper. Writing is a highly sophisticated neurological function. The brain has to take input from reading skills, organize thoughts, apply vision, and use manual dexterity through the movement of the arm and hand—as well as the manipulation of a pencil or pen—into the form of organized, legible writing. This ability is one of the most valuable indicators of excellent brain function. If a child can write well, this confirms that many brain functions are operating on a sophisticated level.

BEHAVIOR CHALLENGES

The behavior challenges that children and teens can exhibit should be categorized between those that are neurological versus those that result from social conditions. Many children labeled as "bad" are not bad at all—they are merely suffering from brain injuries that make them incapable of acting appropriately or demonstrating self-control. When poor behavior is neurologically based, it can result in numerous social and personal development problems and be extremely stressful for the parents and child alike. Parents can experience great confusion, guilt, and even self-recrimination as they wonder if they didn't raise their children well, discipline them enough, or spend enough time with them, all while worrying how they'll be judged by others.

When other developmental challenges accompany poor behavior, disorganization in the brain is the likely culprit. These can be seen as:

- Verbal outbursts
- Tantrums
- Inability to understand and follow boundaries
- Profane language
- Screaming
- Hitting
- Masturbation at a prepuberty age
- Breaking things
- Insubordination to parents or teachers
- Inflicting harm on oneself or others
- Poor eye contact
- Lack of empathy
- Disinterest in working within groups or cultivating friendships
- Little to no motivation to try new things

POOR EMOTIONAL REGULATION

Poor emotions can be displayed by a lack of expression, inappropriate responses (like laughing when someone is sad or injured), or emotions that cannot be controlled or regulated. These symptoms are also frustrating to parents. If a child is continually melancholy or, at the other extreme, prone to regular meltdowns, this could also indicate a brain injury.

SEIZURES

Seizures are an often misunderstood symptom of brain injury. Many people operate under the assumption that seizures cause brain injuries when, in fact, the opposite is true—seizures are the result of brain injuries. A seizure is an attempt by the brain to create a correction—just like a fever is an attempt to kill disease within the body.

All of us experience tiny seizures. A yawn is perhaps the mildest form of seizure. Have you ever been on the verge of falling asleep and your body suddenly jerks or twitches? Technically, this would be considered an extremely mild seizure.

Ultimately, the brain triggers a seizure when it doesn't have enough oxygen. The purpose of a seizure is to increase the oxygen flow to your brain and re-regulate the brain. The pathway that leads to inflammation within the brain (thus lowering oxygen) can stem from a variety of factors, such as cranial pressure, infections, food sensitivities, gut dysfunction, stress and anxiety, overexcitement, and poor function of one or more of the four ventricles in the brain.

When a child or adult has epilepsy due to an injury in the brain, the cause must be identified and treated at the root level.

There are also young children, mostly under age five, who experience febrile seizures triggered by a sudden spike in fever caused by a viral illness like the flu or an ear infection. This type of seizure is usually an isolated incident that is related to the fever, and it rarely results in long-term complications.

Addressing the Symptoms of Seizures

Because seizures are a symptom of brain injury, they are also a symptom of several conditions, most notably epilepsy. Experts in the field of medicine generally do recognize seizures as symptoms, which is good, and traditionally recommend treatments that entail the following conventional methods:

- Limit the threshold and alter the lifestyle/environment to reduce stress
- Medication
- Surgery
- Brain stimulation (vagus nerve stimulator)

Our recommended approach entails these methods:

- Improve cranial motion/flow with cranial-sacral, chiropractic, and other manual therapies
- Neurological stimulation for a more resilient brain
- Improve the nutrition of the brain by looking carefully at diet in terms of food, supplements/vitamins, allergies, bowel health, and elimination
- Physical exercise and good sleep habits
- Increasing blood flow through respiratory therapies

More approaches for addressing specific types of brain injuries will be covered in chapter six.

BRAIN INJURY IS ALL AROUND US

When most people hear the phrase "brain injury," their guts tighten and panic sets in because this is perceived as a terrible, irreversible prognosis. However, over the course of thirty-eight years and working with thousands of children, we've proven beyond a shadow of a doubt that brain injuries are reversible. A brain injury is not something to fear, but rather something to approach with wisdom, precision, and fearlessness.

You and your child are really the same. You have a little of what he or she has a lot of.

So when you wonder or worry over what happened to your child, understand that if he exhibits one or more of the problems noted in this chapter, this is likely due to some form of disorganization or injury within the brain. The reality is that many children have brain injuries—more than most people realize. We would estimate that more than 30 percent of all children have measurable brain injuries that negatively impact their lives. That statistic corresponds with recent Centers for Disease Control (CDC) studies confirming one in six kids have ADD/ADHD, cerebral palsy, Down syndrome, epilepsy, autism spectrum disorders, and other developmental disabilities.

Brain injury is all around us. Our central nervous systems are incredibly complex with many opportunities to go awry. Fortunately, there are just as many opportunities for our brains to heal.

Many kids are coping with their brain injuries. The lucky ones become organized over time. Some are getting by. Some are struggling, and some are in desperate trouble. All of them are in need of healing.

Parents frequently wonder if there is a point at which therapies to heal brain injuries will cease being effective. The good news is that there is no cutoff point. Dr. Marian Diamond, a renowned neuroscientist who once studied the brain of Albert Einstein, conducted groundbreaking research that proved that the anatomy of the brain develops and improves through enrichment, regardless of age, due to brain plasticity.

All of us have an opportunity to become more neurologically capable. There's no reason why, when working with your child, you cannot participate in his progress. All it takes is knowledge, a willingness to work hard, and enough time to make it happen.

FAMILY SUCCESS STORY

We didn't realize our child [Pete] had special needs until he was about twelve years old. He just seemed quirky, and like a very bright young man who just didn't want to do schoolwork and couldn't get along with people. I was embarrassed by his actions most of the time and was getting desperate for help.

My loving friends told me about the Family Hope Center and dragged me to the three-day parent training. At the training, many of the behaviors I'd observed were no longer a mystery. Though I knew this would help my son, I felt like I didn't really belong in the program since my child could walk, talk, and read. Matthew [Newell] acknowledged my concern and told me that many times kids like mine are the most misunderstood and will benefit tremendously from getting organized. Whew! I knew I was in the right place.

Beginning the program was the start of many fights with Pete. The first being the diet. There was a lot of yelling and pushback about the "horrid-tasting food." Every chance he got, he would "cheat" by eating junk. Mostly, all we could accomplish during the first eight months was creeping and crawling, and not nearly the recommended distances. We did our best with where we were. We kept going. Pete needed me.

Even with all the fighting, and the struggle to get all the pieces of the program done, we started seeing progress after about six months. There would be long stretches of time without obvious progress, and then a switch would flip.

We carried a heavy burden of guilt for not helping Pete sooner, for not seeing his needs, and for not being able to do all the program. Yet, we kept at it. Going back for the follow-up visits was crucial for keeping us on track. I needed to be reminded of the brain healing program we were doing. The staff also encouraged me because they could see progress where I was blind to it. They told me I was doing hard work and that Pete was worth it.

Today, Pete is nearing the end of the program, and he is motivated to do it on his own. He's almost eighteen years old and craves his vegetables, often turning down foods on his own and seeking veggies even when we travel.

Without the concerted effort of getting him organized, Pete wouldn't be driving, working, or graduating high school. I'm not worried about him ending up in jail because he exploded at the wrong time. He has friends and will be able to self-regulate in the stresses of life. His anxiety is gone, he has a bright future, and he's a delight.

The program is a gift. The results are priceless.

—*Nellie, Pete's mom*

At the time of this writing, I am seventeen years old. I've been doing this program for just over six years now. And whereas at the start, when I didn't see the point of what I was doing, I now see the benefits. I missed pizza and soda, and a load of other stuff. In short, I *hated* the diet. I hated the exercise.

Now that the end is in sight, and my neurology has pretty much caught up to the best it's going to be, I can say for certain that this program is easily worth its weight in gold. I have friends now. I can react to change, learn, and grow as a person. I'm a better human being.

You're the parent, you make them do it because eventually they will want to as well. Then you'll get to stop pushing. I'm grateful my mom made me do it.

—*Pete*

NEURO-PARENTING POINTS

- The source of most special needs and learning disability diagnosis is a brain injury or impairment.
- Brains become injured in many ways, either before, during, or after birth. These include:
  - gestational conditions
  - birth-related complications
  - traumatic brain injury (TBI)
  - environmental toxins
  - genetics
  - viruses and bacteria
  - stroke

- Brain injuries can be detected through:
    - function
    - blood biochemistry
    - CT scans/MRIs
    - surgery

- Warning signs that indicate probability of a brain injury/impairment in a child include problems with:
    - vision
    - reading
    - attention and focus
    - hearing
    - coordination
    - sensation
    - stuttering
    - language
    - concentration
    - writing
    - behavior
    - emotions
    - seizures

- Brain injury is all around us. The lucky ones became organized. Some are coping or surviving. Some are struggling; some are in deep trouble. Others are desperate.
- The source of the symptoms is the brain injury your child suffered. Once you notice the signs, you can begin to pinpoint dysfunctional areas and develop a comprehensive and tailored strategy toward directly improving the parts of the brain that are compromised.

CHAPTER 4

THE AMAZING BRAIN: HOW IT FUNCTIONS AND GROWS

We're now ready to dig into the parts of the brain and how they work. This will be an informative but packed chapter, so take your time, allowing space to process this information and what it means for your child.

When a child is whole and succeeding, parents often take for granted the magnificence of a well-organized brain that develops, transforms, and adapts over time to learn and grow. Too often, it's only in the agony of watching a child struggle to talk, read, move, connect with others, or feel comfortable in their environment that we search for more knowledge of the brain, seeking a clear solution to the injury that the child is experiencing.

We want you and your family to learn and understand more about the engineering system of the brain. When healthy and functioning well, the brain organizes itself. When it's not well, we need to consistently and thoughtfully implement methods that will help the brain develop and become organized.

Before you can discover and understand how to help your child's brain heal, you first must learn more about various areas of the brain and the functions they control. If one aspect of the brain is not functioning well, it affects the brain overall. Even the seemingly smallest areas of the brain can, if not organized, create havoc for a child. Once you understand more about the brain and brain function, you can begin to assess its efficiency level in your child and then learn how to stimulate it in a manner that will foster improvement and healing.

KEY AREAS OF THE BRAIN

The adult human brain weighs about three pounds and communicates and interrelates with all bodily functions. It is a vital organ that serves as the engineering center for the entire body. The brain receives, processes, and sends thousands of messages per minute to other areas of the body. In short, the brain is the communication center of the nervous system.

The main regions of the brain are the brain stem (consisting of the medulla oblongata, the pons, and midbrain), the limbic system, the cerebellum, and the cerebrum/neocortex. Because successful healing begins with a bottom-up approach, we will introduce these critical areas and their basic/primary functions starting at the base of the brain.

THE BRAIN STEM

At the bottom of the brain lies the brain stem. It connects the spinal cord with the cerebrum, as well as connecting the cerebrum with the cerebellum. The brain stem includes the medulla, the pons, and the midbrain.

The Medulla Oblongata

Nestled at the base of the brain as part of the lower brain stem and connecting with the spinal cord, the medulla oblongata—or "medulla" for short—is responsible for all of the many reflexes hardwired in utero, including the basic infant reflexes such as swallowing and sneezing. It is

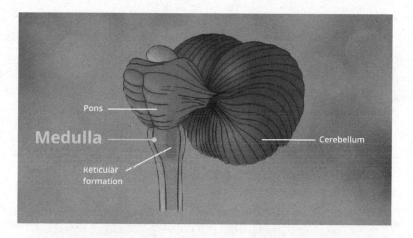

vitally important for this part of the brain to be organized since it maintains the functionality of the respiratory and cardiovascular systems, controls breathing, blood pressure and flow, and heartbeat. The medulla helps infants progress from a basic "survival" stage to the vital and meaningful stages of development.

Injury to the medulla can create severe difficulties—even death—since it is critical to many essential functions in the nervous system, crucial to breathing and heart rate, and is also home to more than twenty infant reflexes.

The Pons

The pons is an incredible part of the brain. It rests above the medulla, and it connects the upper and lower portions of the brain. In fact, in Latin, pons means "bridge." Even though you may be less familiar with it than other parts of the brain, it is important to understand the critical role the pons plays in development.

The pons is vital to the ability to breathe deeply. It controls the facial muscles and the front part of the tongue, which relates to the mechanics of chewing food and managing words. The pons is the messenger of the brain, transmitting messages from the cerebellum and the cerebrum (cerebral cortex). It's responsible for registering and responding to the senses of touch and taste. It immediately reacts to warnings from the body (like "too hot," "too cold," or "that hurts") and the environment (reacting to sounds such as thunder or car horns). This part of the brain also controls tracking with the eyes, a function necessary for reading and catching a ball.

If you look at the images of this baby, you can see the pons in action.

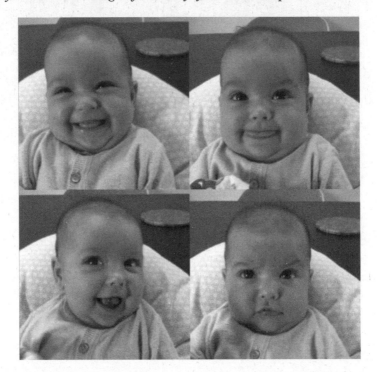

The pons is also the primary home of the essential reticular formation. The reticular formation consists of nerve tracts that run through the brain stem from the medulla through the pons to the midbrain. The reticular formation, among many other things, regulates waking and sleeping, focus, states of consciousness, arousal, and basic self-motivation. It regulates heart and breathing rates, muscle tone, gastrointestinal activity, and bowel and bladder function. The reticular formation also performs tasks that allow a child to stay alert/focused and to filter extraneous noises, important for learning at school and doing homework.

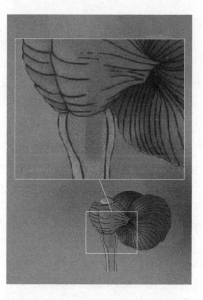

Injury to this part of the brain could result in fatigue, narcolepsy, or even a coma. It can also prevent a child from being able to talk clearly, read across a page, chew, swallow, commando crawl, filter sounds, regulate emotions, focus and pay attention while learning, and respond to vital pains and sounds (like "stop!"). A vast number of school-age children have disorganization in this part of the brain, which makes them prone to distraction and a lack of focus. While a child might be smart and able to recognize many single words, disorganization within the pons can create significant learning and language struggles.

The Midbrain

The midbrain is at the top of the brain stem, below the two cerebral hemispheres. It contains a substantial number of fiber tracts and nerves directly related to vision and eye movement (tracking upward and downward, tracking in circles, and tracking in and out from the face), voluntary muscle activity, and body movement. If injured, there can be problems with vision, hearing, and motor development.

- **Thalamus**
The thalamus is the heart of the brain. It touches and is involved with all primary and sophisticated functions. It is like a router or main sensory relay station and integrative center that connects to many areas of the brain, including the cerebral cortex. It transmits neural impulses to other regions of the brain for processing. The thalamus helps create the foundations for us to think in abstracts such as time, distance, and space, and it supports logical "common sense." Injury to this area of the brain creates many complications for understanding, learning, and coordination. For simplicity, we consider this part of the "midbrain."

- **Hypothalamus**
The hypothalamus is the master control of the autonomic nervous system. This system stimulates and controls structures such as the heart, most glands, and smooth muscles. In effect, it allows the body to excite and relax as needed. The hypothalamus also integrates the endocrine functions and controls hormone production, which regulates growth, metabolism, and reproduction. It also plays a role in influencing bonding behavior and emotional responses. It helps the body recognize hunger and thirst and maintain body temperature. Injury to the hypothalamus can lead to a lack of both emotional and sexual control. For simplicity, we consider this part of the "midbrain."

- **Pineal Body**
This gland-like body is primarily responsible for melatonin production, which helps with sleep and being in harmony with the daily and seasonal rhythms of life. Injury in this area would disrupt circadian rhythms (the natural twenty-four-hour body clock).

- **Basal Ganglia**
The basal ganglia, located within the cerebral hemispheres, are

a group of neurons responsible for motor coordination, refined movement, smooth and even breathing, and remembering repetitive motor tasks. They also control optical convergence to help with depth perception, reading of small print, catching a ball, and walking up and down steps. For simplicity, we consider this part of the "midbrain." Injury to this area can increase the severity of poor muscle tone (rigid or flaccid), inability to refine movements, problems with speech, reading, and comprehension, or understanding the location or source of sounds.

THE LIMBIC SYSTEM

The limbic system is a network of structures within the brain that sits above the midbrain and below the cerebrum. The limbic system houses all our basic emotions and our need to be socially connected with others. The amygdala and the hippocampus are the primary structures of this system. The amygdala is one of two almond-shaped structures leading off the olfactory nerve and the place where emotions like pleasure, anger, and fear are processed. It is linked to the hippocampus, which is primarily responsible for short-term memory, processing and retrieving, and learning. People diagnosed with Alzheimer's, along with possible damage from toxins, have an injury in the limbic system.

The limbic system is always "on" since its primary function is to trigger our instincts and warn us of danger. It controls autonomic functions such as arousal, motivation, emotions, memory, and bonding. The olfactory pathway feeds this part of the brain directly, which affects the sense of smell.

The limbic system also houses the mammillary bodies, which play a role in our conscious and subconscious attitudes about food and episodic memory. This allows us to travel back in time to remember an event that took place at a specific location and time. For example, if you remember the family vacation you took when you were ten, this is an episodic memory.

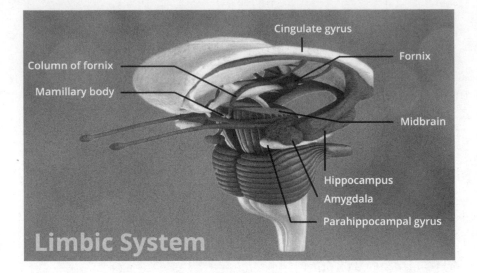

The limbic system also links to the prefrontal cortex, which fosters the ability to interact well with others within multiple social situations. It is the source of emotional intelligence.

Injury to the limbic system results in withdrawal, the avoidance of eye contact and human interaction, and an inability to show empathy for others. It also causes some children to fixate on objects or have difficulty adapting to new situations, which prevents successful integration into social groups.

THE CEREBELLUM

The cerebellum (Latin for "little brain") is located at the back of the head. While not technically part of the midbrain, it does work hand in hand with it. Among its many functions, the cerebellum is primarily responsible for coordinating movement, regulating muscle tone, integrating the motor and sensory pathways, and managing balance, spatial awareness, and equilibrium. Children who have problems in this part of the brain can have difficulty maintaining their balance and muscle coordination. They may experience involuntary movement and speech problems.

THE CEREBRUM

The cerebrum, which is the most substantial part of the brain, consists of two halves—the right and left hemispheres. These hemispheres are connected by nerve fibers (called the corpus callosum) and are in constant communication with each other. The cerebrum, which is made up of both white and gray matter (neocortex), is responsible for learning, thinking, reasoning, language, advanced social behavior, advanced motor skills, and executive function.

Regarding the brain hemispheres, you've probably heard that people who are "right-brained" are creative and those who are "left-brained" are logical. Though that has a bit of truth to it, it is not as much as people think. While the left is primarily responsible for dealing with details, and the right is the big-picture abstract part, both sides work well together. There are some essential differences in the functioning of each hemisphere.

- Right hemisphere (controls the left side of the body):
  - processes information as a whole
  - facilitates nonverbal communication, reading faces and actions
  - moderates emotional intelligence
  - provides comprehension of the "big picture"
  - manages large muscle control for mobility—kinesiology and spatial awareness
  - is responsible for math reasoning
  - interprets information—what does it mean as a whole
  - directs negative emotions—like "be careful" and "avoid this"
  - understands abstract concepts, common sense
  - provides caution and safety—internal warning system; what to avoid versus what is safe

- Left hemisphere (controls the right side of the body):
  - processes information in parts
  - supervises verbal communication—speaking
  - organizes intellectual information

- interprets comprehension of words
- directs small muscle control—writing, ballet, gymnastics, etc.
- enables math calculations
- processes information and analyzes facts
- manages positive emotions—"go for it"
- facilitates linear and logical thinking, sequential commands
- moderates curiosity, impulsivity

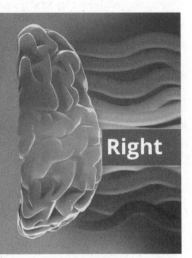

- Processes information as a whole
- Non verbal communication – reading faces and actions
- Emotional intelligence
- Comprehension of big picture
- Large muscle control for mobility – kinesiology – spatial awareness
- Math 'reasoning'
- Interpret information – what does it mean as a whole
- Negative Emotions – avoid / safe
- Understanding abstract concepts –common sense
- Caution and safety – is this ok – warning system

Right

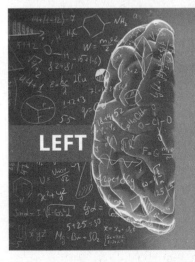

LEFT

- Processes information in parts
- Verbal communication – words
- Intellectual Organization of information
- Comprehension of words
- Small muscle control - i.e. writing – ballet – learning
- Math 'calculations'
- Processing information – analyzing facts
- Positive emotions – go for it
- Linear and logic – sequential commands
- Curious - impulsive

It's interesting to note that the right side of your brain controls the motor activity of the left side of your body, while the left side of your brain controls the right side. However, both hemispheres work together toward both creative and analytical thinking.

The neocortex, located in the upper part of the cortex, like topsoil, is the outer layer and is known as gray matter. It controls many essential functions, including speech and language, information processing, and memory. It is also involved in sensory processing and voluntary muscle movement.

There are four primary parts, or "lobes," of the cerebral cortex.

Frontal Lobe

The frontal lobe is responsible for cognitive function, memory, emotional intelligence, and movement. It consists of three areas:

- *Prefrontal cortex.* This area is responsible for planning, complex ideas, problem-solving, and concentration. It also helps direct and moderate behavioral impulses, emotions, judgment, and inhibition.
- *Primary motor cortex.* This area is responsible for voluntary movement including muscle movement, large muscle motor control, and facial movement.
- *Premotor cortex.* This area is involved in motor planning and the storage of learned motor patterns, which helps guide the direction of movement. It also assists with abstract thinking.

Injury to the frontal lobe can cause difficulties in the processing of speech, critical thinking, social integration, and executive function, as well as challenges with fine motor skills. It can also result in memory problems and a loss of impulse control. Like the limbic system, the prefrontal cortex also helps moderate emotions, and may be unable to restrain unchecked emotions, allowing phobias and panic attacks to emerge, when damaged.

Temporal Lobe

This lobe is primarily responsible for receiving auditory information and recognizing words, which makes it vital to the process of learning and understanding language. It's also involved in regulating sophisticated emotional responses. Other parts of this lobe appear to form, retrieve, and integrate memories including sensory memories of taste, sound, sight, and touch.

Injury to the temporal lobe can impede the ability to process auditory information accurately and other hearing impairments. Damage to this area can also result in overly agitated, irritable, or childish behavior.

Parietal Lobe

This lobe is primarily responsible for processing sensory input and sensory discrimination. It receives and acts on information from the lower levels of the brain about body temperature, taste, touch, movement of the body, and spatial relationships, such as the distance and position of objects.

Injury to the parietal lobe can impair the accuracy of sensory information from the lower levels of the brain. This impairment creates an inability to discriminate between different stimuli (telling the difference between heads and tails of a coin), difficulties in locating and recognizing parts of the body, the inability to write, disorientation in environmental spaces, and problems with self-care.

Occipital Lobe

This lobe is the primary visual center of the brain. It processes information from the eyes and links that information with images stored in memory, which in turn helps you identify what you're looking at.

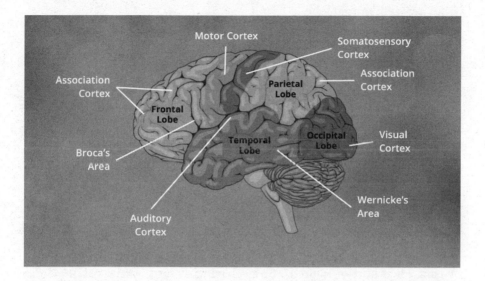

Injury to the occipital lobe can result in visual impairment and, in severe cases, blindness. Damage in this area can also cause hallucinations, make objects appear larger or smaller than they are, and create problems with color recognition.

LEARNING THROUGH THE FIVE SENSES

From the time you're born, whenever you learn something new, the information you receive comes from your five senses. The sensory organs—ears (hearing), eyes (seeing), nose (smelling), skin (touching), and tongue (tasting)—relay this information to the brain. The brain develops remarkably through these sensory experiences during the first few years of life. Babies rely on their senses to learn, engage, and thrive.

As previously noted, each of the senses transmits information from the brain stem to particular cortical areas of the brain for processing:

- Hearing: temporal lobe
- Sight: occipital lobe

- Smell: frontal lobe
- Touch: parietal lobe
- Taste: parietal lobe

An injury to a specific part of the brain will lead to those messages being incorrectly interpreted, if at all. You may notice that everything smells terrible to your child. Or perhaps they're an incredibly picky eater because many foods taste bad or they don't like the texture of the food. Perhaps your child doesn't like the feel of their clothes or dislikes being hugged or touched. Other children may react negatively to loud noises or crowds. These aversions are indicative of disorganization within the brain.

Sometimes, rather than being oversensitive to sensory issues, a child may exhibit signs of being *undersensitive*: not responding to heat, cold, or pain when hurt or injured. Always having to turn up the volume on a television. These types of lacking responses are often due to a hurt brain as well.

Once you identify a sensory issue, you can take steps to foster the connection between the senses and the parts of the brain that are not making those connections. You accomplish this by targeting the root cause of what you see symptomatically in your beloved child.

THE EVER-GROWING, EVER-DEVELOPING BRAIN

Remember neuroplasticity? It's the brain's ability to adapt and change in response to stimulation by establishing new connections in neural pathways. Until recently, it was believed that once we mature from children to adults, the level of our brain's development reaches its peak and then hits a plateau. Therefore, as we gradually approach middle age and the senior years, we are bound to experience a loss of brain cells and some memory lapses, like trouble recalling people's names or remembering where we left the keys.

The good news, however, is that we now know that the brain is more dynamic than we imagined—it has an extraordinary ability to change, adapt, and evolve from the time we take our first breath until our last. Even better news—we can now apply this knowledge to help our children move through their specific challenges.

PHYSIOLOGY VERSUS PATHOLOGY

Physiology is the science of functions and activities of living organisms and their parts. Pathology is the study of disease and its origins. In our terms, physiology deals with working toward developing *normal* biological functions while pathology deals symptomatically with taking away *abnormal* biological functions.

Over the years, illnesses and disabilities have been dealt with through the lens of pathology with the ultimate goal of making right what is wrong to achieve a state of normalcy. Such remedies are as simple as taking an aspirin to alleviate a headache or taking medication to eliminate seizures, reduce heartburn, and increase attention; or as sophisticated as cutting the muscles in a leg to make it less rigid, injecting Botox to weaken a muscle, or cutting the eye muscles to try and correct a convergent or divergent strabismus.

In fact, undertaking various physical therapy techniques, such as wearing braces or ankle-foot orthoses (AFOs), seeks to correct what is showing as a physical issue rather than going to the *source* of the issue—the brain stem. Wearing eyeglasses to pull the eyes inward or outward is a symptom-driven strategy, not a brain strategy. When you take off the glasses, you will see no improvement. If the brain *were* improving from medication, eyeglasses, or braces, the need for these tools would decrease, and the problem would be self-eliminating. But this is not the case.

Medication-based interventions such as muscle relaxers (like baclofen) for brain-injured children seek to alleviate the symptoms but, again, do not address the cause, which is an injury to the brain stem and myofascial dysfunction. Medicating a child for ADHD introduces chemicals into the brain. While that may offer a sense of fixing the problem, it can actually do the opposite, moving further from a solution. Chasing symptoms and not focusing on underlying causes is a dead-end street. There is never a "yes" to this pathological pathway of pursuit.

Pathology says, "Let's suppress or take away the symptoms and maybe things will be better," whereas physiology says, "Let's heal the system and it will self-correct."

As we move forward, we will provide you with neurophysiological and nutritional strategies to help significantly improve the function of your child's brain. That is the difference between a pathological versus a physiological approach.

FUNCTION DETERMINES STRUCTURE

There is a direct connection between function and structure. For example, if you worked out daily, doing sit-ups, push-ups, and weight lifting, you would have toned arms and legs, and your muscles would develop. Depending on your exercise regimen, your body would change overall, and the parts of the body you were working on most would see a marked difference. In other words, the function of exercising would determine the structure of your body.

The opposite is also true—a lack of function will result in a lack of structure. How often have you heard the phrase "use it or lose it"? If you studied French in high school but never practiced speaking it regularly, chances are you gradually forgot what you learned. Similarly, not exercising the body may cause a loss of strength or stamina.

The brain grows by use, and the function of stimulating the brain determines the rate of neuroplasticity. Just as you build your body strength by working out, the same holds true for the brain. When you stimulate the brain, it will grow. For children with brain injuries, stimulating the brain is critical for moving beyond limitations. That's physiology in action.

Brain science is continually evolving, and there are many discoveries yet to be made that will increase our understanding of the amazing brain, how to maintain its health, and how to maximize its potential.

Going forward, the ultimate goal is to understand and address the physiology—via the neurology—of your child's injury and to seek physiological solutions to healing the brain and body. Now that you understand more about the brain, its key areas, and the basic functions each area controls, the next step is to measure and evaluate your child's current physiological status and capabilities.

FAMILY SUCCESS STORY

Edmond was a difficult child since he was one year old. He was intense, but after his first shots at the age of one year and four months, he became unmanageable.

Family members and people around us said it was because of the birth of his little brother, Joseph. Afterward, they blamed "the terrible twos." Then it was because we'd moved to the United States. Inside myself, however, I always knew that something was going on with him.

At school, teachers and parents complained about his behavior, and at home, he was very disruptive and rigid, with unstoppable energy and tantrums. He wanted to eat only sugar, bread, pasta, and cheese. It is sad to say, but Edmond was troublesome. We, as a family, did all we could, and he ended up in a special school with a psychologist, two therapists, a tutor, and a special holistic doctor for well-being.

At the beginning of 2014, my husband, Eddy, and I were running out of hope because we had to try medication as the school requested, with no positive effects. Then our dear friend Florencia recommended we visit the Family Hope Center, a place that helps children with brain injuries.

After the training, the team evaluated Edmond. The result was that he'd had a very severe injury in the whole brain. This was hard to digest, but we believed in the program.

We started working with Edmond in September 2014. We decided to take him out of school and focus on his program. For us, his brain was more important than academics. He spent around seven hours per day, five days a week (and half a day on Saturdays) doing crawling and creeping, working on his reflexes and senses, and doing a lot of breathing exercises. We also bought a hyperbaric chamber, which we used every single day, and we still use it, because it makes you feel great. We were on top of Edmond's diet and vitamins also.

Edmond's brain was healed in approximately three years, and our life changed. We work hard (I must say) with no pause, and a lot of discipline, creativity, and love. We arranged everything so the program was playful for Edmond and me. We laughed, cried, played, fought, and hugged each other a lot.

My heart is full of gratitude for Matt, Carol, and the team at the Family Hope Center for making possible Edmond's transformation and making us a strong and resolute family. Also, for teaching us how to serve our child.

As Antoine de Saint-Exupéry said: "A goal without a plan is just a wish." We had the goal of helping Edmond to have a better life, and the Family Hope Center made a wonderful plan for this to happen.

—*Maria Zambrano, Edmond's mom*

NEURO-PARENTING POINTS

There are several key areas of the brain that are responsible for neurological development.

Brain stem: The brain stem, which connects the cerebrum with the spinal cord, consists of the:

- Medulla oblongata—controls multiple reflexes and maintains functionality of breathing, blood flow, and heart rate.
- The pons—connecting the upper and lower parts of the brain, controls deep breathing, facial muscles, visual tracking, paying attention, bowel and bladder control, self-motivation, and transmits touch and taste sensations, including warning signals.
- The midbrain, which includes:
  - the mesencephalon, which has a role in controlling muscle tone and wherein resides the third and fourth cranial nerves responsible for moving the eyes up and down, in circles and convergence.
  - the thalamus, which relays and integrates sensory information.
  - the hypothalamus, which is the master control of the autonomic nervous system.
  - the basal ganglia, which organizes overall mobility and creates dopamine within one of its structures, the substania nigra.

The Limbic System: Triggers instincts and controls autonomic functions including emotions, motivation, memory, bonding, and sense of smell. The limbic system includes the amygdala (emotional responses) and hippocampus (short-term memory).

Cerebellum: The cerebellum, which is located at the back of the head, is responsible for movement, muscle tone, and balance. Injuries to the cerebellum result in loss of balance and muscle coordination.

Cerebrum: The cerebrum consists of two brain hemispheres connected by the corpus callosum, along with the cerebral cortex. There are four lobes in the cerebral cortex:

- Frontal lobe—controls cognitive function, memory, movement, emotional intelligence. Injury to this lobe results in problems with critical thinking, emotional engagement, and fine motor skills.
- Temporal lobe—controls auditory processing, word recognition, and emotional regulation. Injury to this lobe can lead to hearing-related problems, emotional regulation, and speech.

- Parietal lobe—controls sensory processing and body awareness. Injury to this lobe can lead to problems with the brain/body connection within the environment, math and writing skills, spatial orientation, and self-care.
- Occipital lobe—controls vision and visual memory. Injury in this lobe can result in visual impairment and problems with color recognition.

CHAPTER 5

EVALUATING AND UNDERSTANDING YOUR CHILD'S CAPABILITIES

Dr. Carl Granger, a brilliant medical statistician and executive director of the Center for Functional Assessment Research, aptly stated in a presentation I heard back in 2004: "If you cannot measure it, you cannot manage it."

When you understand where the brain is neurologically, you can then develop a plan to create change. This is your initial reference point. You need to know where you are before you know how to get somewhere.

Too often, professionals evaluate only one ability (like language, vision, or mobility), or even worse, assess a disability and develop programs or treatments to either take away a disability or create a new ability. We think it is vital to evaluate *all* the pathways and areas of the brain and to look at the precious child in a three-dimensional manner. To thoroughly understand the level of anyone's neurological abilities and to accurately develop a strategy to support this process, you need to measure a person's developmental abilities and current levels of proficiency.

To do that, we've studied, reviewed, and researched neurodevelopmental charts from other leaders in the field and added our clinical experience to the mix. The result is the Integrative and Developmental Progression Chart (IDPC). Our point of differentiation is that the IDPC encompasses all the major sensory and motor pathways in relation to the brain—except oral—and can mathematically measure anyone's neurological age, regardless of their chronological age. This comprehensive diagnostic tool assesses brain function across age categories and developmental areas, which will serve as the basis for ongoing measurement of your child's progress.

The IDPC is a valuable tool that provides vital insight into how your child is functioning today and helps to determine the neuro-sequential steps that can and should be taken to create a pathway that promotes neurological growth at all levels of brain function.

Understanding and using the IDPC is critical to helping your child. It is the neurological road map you will follow now that you're in the all-important driver's seat of your child's journey to wellness. Our role at this time is to provide an orientation and guide you through the process.

Please note: What follows is a sweeping overview of the brain and the benchmarks for typical neurological development across various age ranges. This provides general guidance for assessing your child's current neurological status. When parents and professionals take our training courses online or in person, we add more details, nuances, and mathematics, which are covered and addressed together in a classroom setting. However, what you discover by completing the IDPC will enlighten you as to what to strive for, proactively, in your child's development.

ABOUT THE INTEGRATIVE AND DEVELOPMENTAL PROGRESSION CHART: A PROFESSIONAL AND PARENTAL VIEW

As an outpatient orthopedic physical therapist, I have over a decade of experience evaluating patients. I have used various methods to measure and describe a person's range of motion, strength deficits, and functional limitations. In my experience, I have found some assessments to be more helpful than others depending on the patient's challenges.

When my medically complex son was born, I quickly became a pediatric and neurologically based physical therapist out of necessity. We discovered the Family Hope Center and it finally felt like we had direction. Instead of taking a "wait and see" position on how he developed, we had a way to be more proactive, and it was exciting!

Our son was essentially blind at six months of age, and in "visual crisis" as a result of his brain surgery and cranial-nerve eye injury. His neurological level on the chart was 1.55. Fast-forward to today, his neurological level is 25.90 and his vision is his biggest strength.

Understanding the chart allowed us to help him make tremendous progress. We knew what we could do to help him reach the next developmental level. And, more importantly, we knew *why* we had to do it with such frequency, intensity, and duration. It absolutely motivated us and encouraged us to continue even when progress seemed slow.

We utilized the chart to evaluate our older daughter, who was heading toward the diagnosis of ADHD. She would run off while at the zoo and was simply a flight risk who couldn't sit still long enough to color a picture at age four. By "going back" and addressing areas she didn't progress through developmentally, we were able to help her "move forward." The chart helped guide us so we could change the course of her educational experience. She now enjoys sitting to do crafts, artwork, and worksheets, and her kindergarten teacher reports she is a pleasure to have in class.

—*Stephanie Ale, PT, DPT, Cert. MDT, CSCS*

THE FAMILY HOPE CENTER
INTEGRATIVE AND DEVELOPMENTAL PROGRESSION CHART

NAME: _____   DATE OF BIRTH: _____   TODAY'S DATE: _____

BRAIN FUNCTION — SENSORY

BRAIN LEVEL	MEDULLA OBLONGATA • 1	PONS • 2	MIDBRAIN • 3
DEVELOPMENTAL PERIOD	BIRTH TO 0.5 MONTHS	0.5 MONTHS TO 2 MONTHS	2 TO 8 MONTHS
SEEING AND READING	• Display a fast pupil contraction reflex in both eyes	• Find light in a darkened room • See and recognize shapes • Consistently track people and objects	• See and distinguish details from three meters • See changes in facial expression • Bring eyes together and converge vision on an object
HEARING AND UNDERSTANDING	• Display immediate Moro reflex response to a loud and sudden noise • Display immediate, yet controlled, startle reflex response to a repeated loud and sudden noise	• Respond fearfully to a loud and threatening sound, such as thunder, or to a warning cry ("STOP!")	• Recognize and appreciate voice inflection • Quickly hear sounds in environment • Quickly locate source of sounds in environment • Understand significance of familiar sounds • Successfully filter sounds and stay on task • Be at ease in a noisy environment and with all familiar sounds
SENSATION AND TACTILITY	• Display a positive Babinski reflex response while crawling • Display a negative plantar reflex response while walking and a neutral Babinski reflex while supine	• Feel painful/vital sensations, such as cold, hot and a pin or needle, <u>throughout</u> the body • Feel painful/vital sensations <u>instantly</u> throughout the body • Feel painful/vital sensations <u>fully</u>, in terms of intensity, throughout the body	• Feel meaningful sensations, such as light touch, stroking, kissing, tickling, warm and cool temperatures, <u>throughout</u> the body • Feel meaningful sensations <u>instantly</u> throughout the body • Feel meaningful sensations <u>fully</u> throughout the body

CHRONOLOGICAL AGE: _____   INITIAL CHRONOLOGICAL AGE: _____

NEUROLOGICAL AGE: _____   INITIAL NEUROLOGICAL AGE: _____

CORTEX • 4	CORTEX • 5	CORTEX • 6	CORTEX • 7	CORTEX • 8
8 TO 12 MONTHS	12 TO 18 MONTHS	18 TO 36 MONTHS	36 TO 72 MONTHS	CHRONOLOGICAL AGE LEVEL
• See in three dimensions, perceiving depth • Begin to have far-point depth perception	• Perceive pictures as abstract representations of concrete objects	• Recognize and identify numerals • Recognize and identify letters of the alphabet	• Read at least 50 single words and simple phrases	• Read in content and speed as well as peers • Demonstrate uniform hemispheric dominance (Age _____)
• Understand at least ten common words and basic couplets • Understand/follow simple requests • Remember simple events and familiar people • Understand basic time concepts, such as "wait" and "in a moment"	• Understand at least 50 words, as well as phrases and simple sentences • Understand/follow a simple two-step request • Understand the time relationships of a typical day	• Understand thousands of words and simple paragraphs • Understand/follow a basic three-step request • Understand basic time concepts, such as yesterday, today, and tomorrow • Understand basic spatial concepts, such as underneath, on top of, and around	• Understand complex paragraphs and stories • Follow a common four-step request • Understand/follow basic concepts in organized games • Understand simple mathematical concepts • Safely remain alone for short periods	• Understand sophisticated life concepts and relationships as well as peers • Demonstrate uniform hemispheric dominance (Age _____)
• Feel the dynamic tactile relationships in three-dimensional objects	• Locate a favorite toy by feel with each hand, without looking	• Feel and identify an object by its physical characteristics (hard, soft, round, flat) with each hand	• Feel the difference between sophisticated and similar objects, e.g., can determine the difference between two sides of a coin, with each hand	• Demonstrate uniform hemispheric dominance (Age _____)

BRAIN LEVEL	MEDULLA OBLONGATA • 1	PONS • 2	MIDBRAIN • 3
DEVELOPMENTAL PERIOD	BIRTH TO 0.5 MONTHS	0.5 MONTHS TO 2 MONTHS	2 TO 8 MONTHS
LOCOMOTION AND MOBILITY	• Display an immediate asymmetrical tonic neck reflex in the supine position • Display an immediate tonic neck reflex when placed in the prone position	• Independently crawl on stomach across the floor one meter • Independently crawl as a means of transportation • Independently crawl in an unrestricted and coordinated pattern	• Independently creep on hands and knees across the floor three meters • Independently creep on hands and knees as a means of transportation • Independently creep on hands and knees in an unrestricted and coordinated cross pattern
COMMUNICATION AND SPEECH	• Demonstrate an initial birth cry • Cry to express needs, such as hunger, tiredness, pain, and discomfort	• Cry in response to pain and distress • Cry loud enough to be heard and rescued	• Create many different sounds to relay emotions and needs, such as happy, hungry, and tired • Create a full range of vowel and consonant sounds
MANUAL AND WRITING	• Reflexively grasp an object placed in hands • Have a strong grasp reflex in both hands	• Release an object from each hand, quickly and completely, when in pain or danger	• Reach out and grab an object with a prehensile grasp with each hand • Release an object voluntarily from each hand • Pass an object from one hand to the other • Begin feeding using own hands
EMOTIONAL AND SOCIAL — LIMBIC BRAIN	• Be comforted by touch, sound, or smell • Accept and seek security	• Adjust to daily routine • Express needs with various cries • Show attention to people and the environment	• Show interest in and interact with parents • Begin to seek affection • Display curiosity and begin to explore environment, consistent with locomotion • Recognize when a familiar object disappears • Communicate with reciprocated facial and vocal expression

BRAIN FUNCTION

MOTOR

SOCIAL

CORTEX • 4	CORTEX • 5	CORTEX • 6	CORTEX • 7	CORTEX • 8
8 TO 12 MONTHS	12 TO 18 MONTHS	18 TO 36 MONTHS	36 TO 72 MONTHS	CHRONOLOGICAL AGE LEVEL
• Independently and consistently walk three meters across the room using the arms for balance	• Stand up in the middle of the floor independently and walk three meters, without using arms for balance • Walk as a means of transportation in an unrestricted and coordinated cross pattern	• Independently run ten meters nonstop • Independently run in an unrestricted and coordinated cross pattern • Hop in place on one foot	• Independently and bilaterally hop across a room five meters nonstop	• Become proficient in new physical challenges as quickly as peers • Learn new physical skills as quickly as peers • Demonstrate uniform hemispheric dominance (Age _____)
• Voluntarily communicate with four meaningful words/signs that are understood by parents	• Voluntarily communicate with 20 meaningful single words/signs • Voluntarily communicate with at least three meaningful couplets using words/signs	• Voluntarily put a meaningful, organized sentence together • Voluntarily tell a meaningful, organized short story • Speak as clearly as peers	• Voluntarily use organized paragraphs to express ideas • Sequentially express information, as in a short story, event, or movie	• Voluntarily speak and express ideas as well as peers (Age _____)
• Cortically oppose thumb and finger in each hand • Begin feeding self using a utensil • Hold a cup and drink from it	• Use both hands together, cortically opposing the thumb and finger • Build structures using blocks • Begin basic dressing and undressing—taking off socks/shoes	• Use hands for sophisticated skills (button, zip, screw), as quickly and easily as peers • Dress and undress using one hand in a lead role • Pour liquid using one hand in a lead role	• Draw people with distinct body parts • Voluntarily write ten words • Voluntarily write five couplets • Write clearly	• Write organized sentences • Write organized paragraphs • Write thoughts spontaneously and voluntarily as well as peers • Write clearly • Demonstrate uniform hemispheric dominance (Age _____)
• Participate in interactive play • Seek parents, objects when moved out of sight • Start to imitate behavior • Assert position; begin to test boundaries • Experiment with a variety of objects • Transition smoothly from one situation to another	• Make good eye contact while communicating including joint attention • Express wide range of emotions appropriately • Play alongside other children (parallel play) with adult support • Engage in purposeful activities	• Recognize link between behaviors and consequences • Share toys and play with others (supervised) • Engage in fantasy games and role-playing to express emotion and concept formation • Spontaneously help others • Refer to self using "me" or "I" • Feel and display remorse and pride	• Work with others, and seek opportunities to solve problems for the family • Engage in a team or group setting and follow the rules of the group • Modify behavior to achieve a positive outcome and/or avoid a negative outcome • Begin to gain insight into possible causes of emotions	• Consider thoughts, needs, and emotions of others • Engage in group activities with peers independently • Defer gratification • Develop meaningful and appropriate relationships • Self-motivated to meet own needs and others' needs (Age _____)

USING THE IDPC

The IDPC outlines the neurotypical benchmarks for sensory, motor, and emotional/social skills among the following seven areas of brain function:

- Seeing and Reading
- Hearing and Understanding
- Sensation and Tactility
- Locomotion and Mobility
- Communication and Speech
- Manual and Writing
- Emotional and Social

Eight developmental levels, starting at birth and through six years of age and beyond, are progressed through in each area.

Because children who are neurologically impaired have wide and varied degrees of functionality, you might find, for example, that your five-year-old's level of communication and speech meets the abilities of a two-year-old. Intellectually, this discovery can confirm what you have already observed about your child, but emotionally, this reality could evoke a sense of sadness, loss, or pain. This response is common and is entirely natural and justifiable. If you find yourself overcome with emotion, we encourage you to take a moment to breathe. Further, do not lose sight of the purpose of this process: to measure your child's *abilities*. By understanding and confirming all the functions and skills your child has *today*, you can focus on helping develop or improve those functions. Use what you learn as the starting point on the road map for your child's journey to healing. As you go through this evaluation process, stay focused on the goal, and remain positive—remember, you are being given a detailed view into what is going on in your child's brain, which is both enlightening and promising.

By recording the level of your child's abilities and consequently measuring the brain's function, you can then create a customized plan of treatment—the road map—that will "move" your child across the chart to successive levels of brain function.

Placing your child's abilities within our IDPC matrix allows you to see "future functioning" as a goal and is a significant way to involve you in your child's developmental process.

MEASURING THE BRAIN

To begin, let's explore each of the eight age-related developmental levels so you can better understand what should be happening in the brain. To make this easier, we've created worksheets with charts to guide you through the process. At each developmental level, note how proficient your child is in each area of brain function by recording your assessments of their current function in the boxes of the right column. You can abbreviate as follows:

A	Achieved (Always)
NA	Nearly Achieved (Most of the time)
PA	Partially Achieved (Sometimes)
NYA	Not Yet Achieved (Little to not at all yet)

You will assign a value to *each bullet* listed. When done, your chart should look something like the chart on the following page.

You will record your responses for each of the eight age levels until all the levels are complete. Each section that follows will include a blank chart that corresponds to an applicable developmental level. After evaluating each area at each level, you'll be able to see a comprehensive overview of your child's neurological status, including which areas need more attention and concentration.

BRAIN LEVEL	MEDULLA OBLONGATA • 1 BIRTH TO 2 WEEKS	YOUR CHILD'S SCORE
SEEING AND READING	• Display a fast pupil contraction reflex in both eyes	A
HEARING AND UNDERSTANDING	• Display immediate Moro reflex response to a loud and sudden noise • Display immediate, yet controlled, startle reflex response to a repeated loud and sudden noise	PA
SENSATION AND TACTILITY	• Display a positive Babinski reflex response while crawling • Display a negative plantar reflex response while walking and a neutral Babinski reflex while supine	NA
LOCOMOTION AND MOBILITY	• Display an immediate asymmetrical tonic neck reflex in the supine position • Display an immediate tonic neck reflex when placed in the prone position	NA
COMMUNICATION AND SPEECH	• Demonstrate an initial birth cry • Cry to express needs, such as hunger, tiredness, pain, and discomfort	A
MANUAL AND WRITING	• Reflexively grasp an object placed in hands • Have a strong grasp reflex in both hands	NA
EMOTIONAL AND SOCIAL LIMBIC BRAIN	• Be comforted by touch, sound, or smell • Accept and seek security	NA

LEVEL 1: BIRTH TO TWO WEEKS

Remember what you read in the previous chapter about the anatomy of the brain? Here's where you get to delve inside and see those parts in action in your child. Some lights will burn brightly, while others will be faint or off.

Do you recall the medulla oblongata? It's the part of the brain that runs all the basic reflexes. When a baby is born, the medulla is ready to fire up its associated reflexes. The medulla controls at least twenty reflexes, but for the purposes of our evaluative chart, we've narrowed it down to the most essential.

SEEING AND READING

Light reflex is the ability for the eyes to dilate and constrict quickly and responsively to different levels of illumination. Babies are born with an imperfect light reflex as they have mainly been in darkness for nine months. After a few weeks of normal day-to-day life, the brain develops the ability for the eyes to constrict and dilate well to light stimulation, and the reflex is now automatic and operating correctly.

HEARING AND UNDERSTANDING

During the first few months of life, if something bangs or crashes, or you loudly clap your hands near a baby, the child will become startled aurally or even cry. This is the startle reflex (also called *Moro reflex*) in action. By the time the baby is two or three months old, he may respond to the sound with a sudden blink. If he is startled, it should happen initially, but not when you clap a second or third time.

A reaction to loud noise is common and indicative of functional hearing. If, after a time, the baby continues to persistently startle, or if any sudden sound like a cough or sneeze makes his body jump, the lack of integration of this auditory reflex tells us that the medulla isn't functioning as it should.

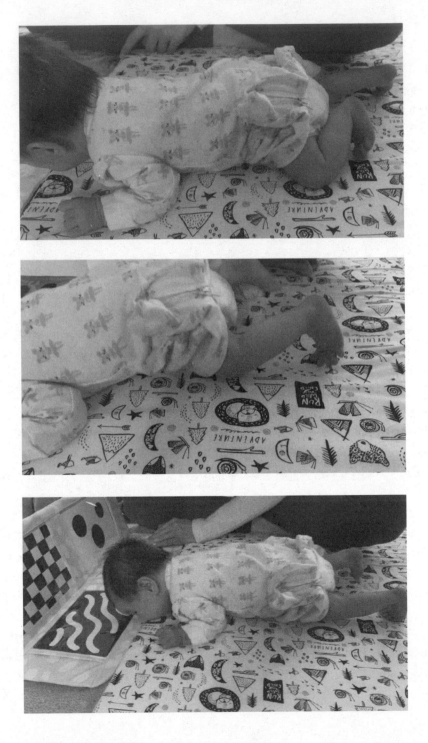

SENSATION AND TACTILITY

If you put a newborn baby in the prone (stomach down) position on the floor, the baby will try to move by pushing off with his big toe and, eventually, commando crawl. This response is called the *Babinski reflex*. Babies desperately need this reflex to crawl. The Babinski reflex is necessary for early movement and should remain throughout life. If you were to commando crawl, you would be using your feet and toes to push off, as depicted in the images on the previous page of an infant attempting just that.

Once a child is walking, this reflex should be neutral when the child is supine. When a child is starting to walk, the toes, as a reflex, need to be going down and gripping the floor, not turning up. This is called a *plantar reflex*. It would be difficult to walk or maintain balance when walking if the toes turned up. If this occurs, and the child can't walk uphill or downhill, it may be perceived as a balance issue when it's actually a reflex issue.

Ninety percent of the children we see in our practice have dysfunction in this part of the brain and this pathway. The Babinski reflex and the plantar reflex, which are two sides of the same coin, play a vital role in the ability to crawl, walk, and balance, linking up with other major reflexes to support ankle, hip, spine, and shoulder function. When not functioning correctly, other reflexes of the medulla, such as the tendon guard, trunk extension, cross leg flexion, the spinal galant, spinal perez, and the headrighting reflex, cannot activate together in a synchronized fashion.

LOCOMOTION AND MOBILITY

When you place a baby on her back, she is going to move her head to one side while extending the arm and leg on that side in the same direction. This action is called the *asymmetrical tonic neck reflex*, which is a primitive reflex that's present at birth. This reflex helps a baby to make its way through the birth canal when being born. This is a water reflex—remember, your baby was in water for nine months before birth. Even while sleeping on the back, most of us will extend the arm in the same direction our head is turned.

However, when you place a baby on her stomach (prone position), she should naturally turn her head toward the flexed upper limb, as shown in the following image. This is called the *tonic neck reflex*.

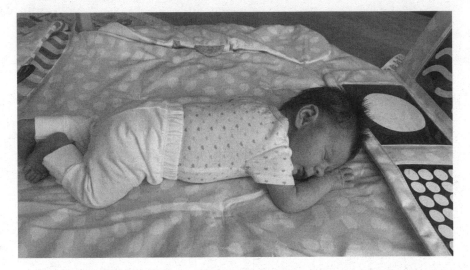

The tonic neck reflex is the "king" of all reflexes because it leads to independent, cross-pattern movement of all the limbs and eventually toward commando crawling and then creeping on the hands and knees.

VAGINAL AND C-SECTION BIRTHS TO EARLY NEUROLOGICAL DEVELOPMENT

In an uncomplicated vaginal birth, a baby starts life with several unique advantages. First, as a baby makes its way through the birth canal, it swallows some of its mother's birth fluid, which contains microbacteria that are healthy to the baby because they help the intestines quickly develop the microbiome to digest food. The large intestine produces 50 percent of the neurotransmitters in the brain. Without this transfer of bacteria, it could take up to six months for the baby to get the necessary microbiome to enhance digestion and maintain its flow.

Second, contractions of the mother's uterus stimulate the reflexes and motion necessary to move a baby down through the birth canal. As the baby emerges through the birth canal, the compression and then expansion of the head, when released into the world, create the first post-birth craniosacral motion, which in turn supports development.

Third, as a baby travels down the birth canal, it also smells its mother in the most profound way, creating a unique sensory/olfactory limbic system link between the baby and its mother. This helps take the baby from an intense sympathetic nervous system experience to a relaxed parasympathetic nervous system experience, especially when a newborn baby is placed against the mother's body after birth.

This brilliant, primordial connection is lost or delayed during a C-section. This sensory connection—or lack thereof—at birth can potentially make a difference to the child's early development.

Of course, C-sections are often a medical necessity. A complication may arise during the birth process that could compromise the health and well-being of the baby or the mother. When precious lives are at stake, mothers are rushed into surgery to minimize or avoid any risks, and their babies are born, within moments, to great relief.

COMMUNICATION AND SPEECH

At birth, all babies cry or should cry. It's a declaration of independence. They're neither happy nor sad; they're just announcing: "I'm here." They've emerged out of the womb and into the world. Think about how you felt when you first heard the sound of your child.

Later, whenever your baby wakes up from a nap, they'll cry to get your attention or their needs addressed. Initially, the cry means they want to be noticed, picked up, and secured. Once the pons engages, a cry can indicate hunger or discomfort.

MANUAL AND WRITING

Raise your hands in the air and make a fist in each. Look at your fists and the position of your thumbs. With hope, your thumbs are across the other three bent fingers as shown in the image below. This is what a well baby's hands look like, too. All babies are born with a neurologically hardwired grasp reflex. Most babies will move their hands in and out of the grasp reflex position often for a few weeks after birth. If you touch their hand, they will grasp your finger tightly.

This reflex is always with you, meaning you'll automatically grab objects with a full, complete grip. A thumb constantly lying alongside or inside the fist may point to dysfunction of the manual pathway.

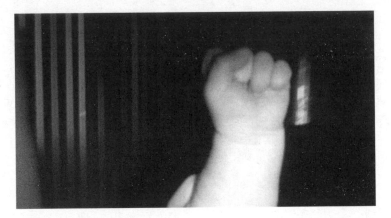

EMOTIONAL AND SOCIAL

The limbic system controls emotional and social behavior. When your child is born, they should be comforted by your smell, your touch, and your presence. Your child should also seek and accept security. If your baby cries, and you pick them up and comfort them, they should regulate and respond to you through your familiar voice, touch, and smell. Make a note of the extent to which your child responds to your gestures of comfort when holding him.

Some children cry constantly and are difficult to comfort. Mothers and fathers can become frustrated because they think they are inadequate at comforting the child, but this can absolutely be a result of limbic disorganization or injury. Some children are "too good" and never cry out for anything, but babies should *always* be announcing they are awake—in need of security and nourishment. The root of the limbic system is the olfactory pathway—the sense of smell. Children and adults should have a balanced sense of smell. Some children are hypersensitive or hyposensitive to smell and this will affect their emotions, bonding, regulation, and the foods they will eat.

BRAIN LEVEL	MEDULLA OBLONGATA • 1 BIRTH TO 2 WEEKS	YOUR CHILD'S SCORE
SEEING AND READING	• Display a fast pupil contraction reflex in both eyes	
HEARING AND UNDERSTANDING	• Display immediate Moro reflex response to a loud and sudden noise • Display immediate, yet controlled, startle reflex response to a repeated loud and sudden noise	
SENSATION AND TACTILITY	• Display a positive Babinski reflex response while crawling • Display a negative plantar reflex response while walking and a neutral Babinski reflex while supine	
LOCOMOTION AND MOBILITY	• Display an immediate asymmetrical tonic neck reflex in the supine position • Display an immediate tonic neck reflex when placed in the prone position	
COMMUNICATION AND SPEECH	• Demonstrate an initial birth cry • Cry to express needs, such as hunger, tiredness, pain, and discomfort	
MANUAL AND WRITING	• Reflexively grasp an object placed in hands • Have a strong grasp reflex in both hands	
EMOTIONAL AND SOCIAL LIMBIC BRAIN	• Be comforted by touch, sound, or smell • Accept and seek security	

LEVEL 2: TWO WEEKS TO TWO MONTHS

The period between the ages of two weeks and two months is when the pons area (which houses most of the reticular formation) of the brain stem kicks in. The pons is the vital part of the brain and basically acts as a messenger of the brain, transmitting information upward from the medulla and to and from the cerebellum, limbic system, and cerebrum. The pons is vigilant and constantly registering and responding to the environment. At this point in neurotypical infant development, the brain is constantly taking in new information as it's aroused by light, sound, and touch.

SEEING AND READING

In addition to light, at this stage babies begin noticing and tracking familiar shapes, objects, and people. If you walk past the crib, your baby's eyes will follow you. The same goes for holding up a bottle—babies will follow that familiar object with their eyes. These actions demonstrate the pons at work, helping the eyes to find the light and shadows automatically and recognize and follow people and objects. The ability to track with the eyes is necessary for peripheral vision and security, learning to read, finding a toy in a playroom, scanning an environment, and so on—it's a vital skill used all day.

HEARING AND UNDERSTANDING

When you hear a sudden loud and threatening noise, like the blare of a truck horn or roar of thunder, you probably jump and have a tinge of fear. If you heard the blare of a fire alarm or air-raid siren, you would probably get up and run to a safe place, right? That is normal and good! That's the pons going into action. We use our hearing to track sounds—that fire alarm compels us to move in the direction of safety, to an exit. This response mechanism is already in action, in babies and children, at the most basic level. If you loudly call out "Stop!" to a small child because they're about to touch something hot, chances are their body will freeze momentarily and then they will start to cry.

Having an immediate response to a sudden, intense sound is vital because it is part of an internal warning system that helps children protect themselves from danger as they grow.

SENSATION AND TACTILITY

The ability to perceive pain is necessary because it protects us from further injury. If you touch something hot, cold, or sharp, you pull away from whatever is causing an unpleasant or painful sensation to the skin and body. The reaction is the same when experiencing the pressure of bumping into something or falling, or the bodily sensation caused by a stomachache or an earache. When these things happen to a child, sometimes they will react and cry immediately; other times, they will become unsettled and in need of a moment to process and breathe before the cry occurs. For a child too disorganized to communicate pain or discomfort, such as when experiencing a stomachache or toothache, the response might be to make a face of pain and cry.

When you observe your child, make a note of the way in which they respond to any sense of pain. The response should be immediate and fully felt.

LOCOMOTION AND MOBILITY

The ability to commando crawl (moving on the belly) starts at birth when babies, if given the opportunity, will move up to the mother's breast and nurse. If you place your baby on a smooth, firm, and warm surface, in most cases, the baby will begin to activate the tonic neck reflex and Babinski reflex to move on their stomach.

The pons is responsible for commando crawling. The primary reflexes are, in a sense, responsible for jump-starting independent crawling.

Crawling is a *vital* part of human development—not just for mobility but also in firing up neurons that manage many other functions. (We will cover this in detail in chapter six.) In fact, the cranial nerves coming out of the pons govern facial muscles used for communication and chewing, as well as the eye muscle (lateral rectus) for tracking. Crawling is *essential* in developing these abilities.

When babies and infants are overcoming the effects of gravity and developing the ability to crawl, you should see the tonic neck reflex in full expression—a beautiful thing to witness. The arms work in coordination—homolateral and then evolving to cross-lateral coordination—with the feet, legs, and head moving to the flexed upper limb, creating a fluid motion.

COMMUNICATION AND SPEECH

Crying is a vital way in which children communicate. Vocalization is necessary to express needs and indicate pain or distress and, in babies, this is accomplished through crying. If your child is in trouble or distress and needs attention, he needs to cry loud enough so that you can hear and attend to him. Evaluate if your child's current cry is loud enough to be heard through the home for him to be rescued.

MANUAL AND WRITING

During the first few weeks of life, babies have a natural and robust grasp reflex. By the time they reach two months of age (engaging the pons), they can release a grasp when in pain. It is vital to have this ability if there is any pain or discomfort. If you picked up the metal handle of a hot pan, your hand would automatically release the item. The same goes for babies. If they grasp the end of something sharp, hot, or cold, they should be able to release the object immediately to avoid further danger or pain. If they do, it indicates that the pons is working correctly. If they do not, and the hand tightens around the object or the release is delayed, this could indicate dysfunction in the manual pathway. Sometimes one hand is performing well and the other not. If so, indicate this.

EMOTIONAL AND SOCIAL

At this level, there are three things to monitor:

- Is your child adjusted to a daily routine? Do they wake at a reasonable hour? Do they sleep well at night? Do they nap regularly? Do they have a good feeding routine? Are you able to reasonably predict when these pivotal moments will occur? If your child is lacking a regular daily eating and sleep cycle, this indicates they haven't adapted neurologically to a routine. If they have any difficulty adjusting to a change in their routine, take note as this could affect how they adapt to transitions in routine over time.
- Does your child express their needs with various cries? Not just in the physical ability to vocalize, but also in the ability to communicate their emotional needs. Babies are actually aware of and attentive to the environment—you can even see when they're tuned in to what's going on. Does your child let you know if they are lonely, hungry, tired, and has needs? Some children do not have certain needs, and parents must account for this daily.
- Does your child focus attention on people and the immediate environment? Socially, babies at this stage may not yet be interacting with others, but they are very aware of their caretakers and parents. You can see in their faces how their emotional states change based on what's going on around them. You may notice their awareness of whatever is close by as well as a response to motion and sound.

BRAIN LEVEL	PONS • 2 2 WEEKS TO 2 MONTHS	YOUR CHILD'S SCORE
SEEING AND READING	• Find light in a darkened room • See and recognize shapes • Consistently track people and objects	
HEARING AND UNDERSTANDING	• Respond fearfully to a loud and threatening sound, such as thunder, or to a warning cry ("STOP!")	
SENSATION AND TACTILITY	• Feel painful/vital sensations, such as cold, hot, and a pin or needle, <u>throughout</u> the body • Feel painful/vital sensations <u>instantly</u> throughout the body • Feel painful/vital sensations <u>fully</u>, in terms of intensity, throughout the body	
LOCOMOTION AND MOBILITY	• Independently crawl on stomach across the floor one meter • Independently crawl as a means of transportation • Independently crawl in an unrestricted and coordinated pattern	
COMMUNICATION AND SPEECH	• Cry in response to pain and distress • Cry loud enough to be heard and rescued	
MANUAL AND WRITING	• Release an object from each hand, quickly and completely, when in pain or danger	
EMOTIONAL AND SOCIAL LIMBIC BRAIN	• Adjust to daily routine • Express needs with various cries • Show attention to people and the environment	

LEVEL 3: TWO TO EIGHT MONTHS

This is the age group in which we begin to see activity in the midbrain. During midbrain development (mesencephalon/thalamus/basal ganglion), the environment starts to become meaningful to the child. Ideally, this part of the brain should be well organized by eight months of age and continue functioning optimally throughout life. When children are hurt, however, brain-stem abilities will require stimulation to develop properly. Once the brain becomes organized, the overall organization of the child will flourish.

SEEING AND READING

If you recall, visually the pons controls the cranial nerves responsible for moving the eyes from side to side. During the development of the midbrain, cranial nerves III (oculomotor) and IV (abducen) begin to engage and create the ability to move the eyes up and down, in circles, and in and out. These cranial nerves work with specific muscles (inferior and superior oblique rectus) to help the eyes function together and to converge the vision on a single object. These abilities lay the foundation for depth perception at far point and near point.

The midbrain is also responsible for noticing details in the face so that babies can now see and recognize their mother and father, as well as detecting changes in a parent's facial expressions—smiles and frowns—both close-up and at three meters (about ten feet). Babies can also respond to facial expressions they see in others, so that if a friend or neighbor smiles and coos at them, they will reciprocate.

Babies can also bring their eyes together in a well-coordinated manner so that they see one converged image. This initiates basic depth perception. If you notice your child displaying a convergent or alternating convergent strabismus or divergent strabismus, this developmentally correlates to disorganization within the midbrain. If your child has strabismus (an eye turning in or out) you may see them turn their head slightly to the side to reduce the double vision to one image.

HEARING AND UNDERSTANDING

Between two and eight months, a child becomes more neurologically organized and able to hear everything, be tuned in to everything, respond to everything, and pay attention to people and the immediate environment. Your child should have the ability to recognize familiar sounds because those sounds now have meaning. They should be generally comfortable with all environmental sounds such as the vacuum cleaner, blender, and dishwasher.

At this point, the child is comfortable in a noisy environment and can filter relevant sounds (the voices of family members, for example) against the background noise. You'll also notice that your child can understand, distinguish, and respond to vocal inflections, picking up tones of affection, seriousness, sadness, or disapproval from Mom or Dad.

Responses to sound are now more immediate. How quickly does your child hear and respond to what you say? Does he know exactly where a sound is coming from and is he able to locate it? For example, if you speak while standing behind your child, do his eyes and head turn to find you? A child should be completely tuned in to every sound in a room and know how to converge the hearing in his ears to locate it.

Your child should also be able to enter a noisy environment, filter out and adjust to the sounds, and not be disturbed by them. These are essential skills because, as they mature, children need to filter out and not become distracted by background noises or irrelevant sounds. Having this ability is necessary for concentration and focus. If this is not the case, the auditory pathway can shut down, which poses a different set of challenges. Any deviation from the above norm—misunderstanding of sounds or inflection, hyper- or hyposensitivity to sounds, inability to locate in direction, or a need to use white noise to calm themselves—is an indication of disorganization in this pathway.

SENSATION AND TACTILITY

A meaningful sensation is the ability to feel different touches and textures. Children at this stage now enjoy being kissed on the belly button, being tickled, cuddled, or having a warm bath. They should be comfortable with body sensations. Others may have the opposite response—being irritated by an item of clothing or the label in a shirt, shoes being too confining, or crying if you clean their face, or brush their hair or teeth.

Children who are hypersensitive or even hyposensitive or do not feel brushes on their body, and don't respond with giggles to kisses, or soften up to light touch, are demonstrating that they are disorganized in this pathway.

Take notice of how your child responds to sensations like a kiss, a tickle, a shoulder rub, or hair stroking. Gauge the response you receive. Is it verbal or is it a stiff or uncomfortable nonverbal reaction shown in the body? Do they overreact, underreact, or feel comfortable by these actions?

LOCOMOTION AND MOBILITY

At the previous level (level two, the pons level), if given a good, healthy amount of opportunity, children begin commando crawling on their stomach. When they reach the midbrain here at level three, they push up, defy gravity, rock back and forth using the asymmetrical tonic neck reflex, and are at the point of creeping on hands and knees. When creeping, the hands should be nice and straight, and the arms and shoulders should help support the hands. Children should be able to creep independently on hands and knees, moving from one place to another as a means of transportation, in a coordinated pattern for three meters (about ten feet). You may also notice your child gaining awareness of personal space (the beginning of dynamic depth perception) as he transports himself by creeping and exploring everywhere throughout the house.

COMMUNICATION AND SPEECH

Before children can speak words, they start by vocalizing many meaningful sounds—these convey needs or moods such as being happy, tired, curious, hungry, or annoyed. They may babble or create the type of sounds you hear in speech or language. Your trained ear and knowledge of your child's mood will help translate and connect the sounds with their needs and emotions—a happy, playful sound is entirely different from one expressing hunger.

When you're with your child, listen carefully. Does she babble most of the day with a nice variety of sounds? Or does she babble only part of the day and have more extended periods of quiet? Pay attention to the frequency and range of sounds she makes.

When listening to these utterances, do you hear vowel and consonant sounds forming, like *a, e, i, o, b, d, m, n, s, ch, k,* and so on? If so, do these sounds correspond only to expressions of emotion or to all vocalizations?

This is the stage where you will recognize the early stages of verbal communication and the roots of language development.

MANUAL AND WRITING

In manual ability, first comes the grasp reflex. Next is the ability to let go and release an object when it causes pain. Now, the hands are being used in a more meaningful way. A child can pick up an object with either hand or transfer an object from one hand to the other. She can intentionally let go of the object when she wants to put it down or drop it voluntarily. A child can also pick up an object, like a toy or piece of food, and put it in her mouth. There's a definite progression in how the hands are now being used. If your child is slow and uncoordinated while attempting to pick up an object, or capable using one hand but not the other hand, this would indicate disorganization in this pathway.

BRAIN LEVEL	MIDBRAIN • 3 2 TO 8 MONTHS	YOUR CHILD'S SCORE
SEEING AND READING	• See and distinguish details from three meters • See changes in facial expression • Bring eyes together and converge vision on an object	
HEARING AND UNDERSTANDING	• Recognize and appreciate voice inflection • Quickly hear sounds in environment • Quickly locate source of sounds in environment • Understand significance of familiar sounds • Successfully filter sounds and stay on task • Be at ease in a noisy environment and with all familiar sounds	
SENSATION AND TACTILITY	• Feel meaningful sensations, such as light touch, stroking, kissing, tickling, warm and cool temperatures, throughout the body • Feel meaningful sensations instantly throughout the body • Feel meaningful sensations fully throughout the body	
LOCOMOTION AND MOBILITY	• Independently creep on hands and knees across the floor three meters • Independently creep on hands and knees as a means of transportation • Independently creep on hands and knees in an unrestricted and coordinated cross pattern	
COMMUNICATION AND SPEECH	• Create many different sounds to relay emotions and needs, such as happy, hungry, and tired • Create a full range of vowel and consonant sounds	
MANUAL AND WRITING	• Reach out and grab an object with a prehensile grasp with each hand • Release an object voluntarily from each hand • Pass an object from one hand to the other • Begin feeding using own hands	
EMOTIONAL AND SOCIAL LIMBIC BRAIN	• Show interest in and interact with parents • Begin to seek affection • Display curiosity and begin to explore environment, consistent with locomotion • Recognize when a familiar object disappears • Communicate with reciprocated facial and vocal expression	

EMOTIONAL AND SOCIAL

At this level, babies begin showing interest in interacting with parents face-to-face. They listen to what Mom or Dad is saying and look and respond to their facial expressions. In fact, babies communicate with reciprocal expressions. They notice when you smile and respond in kind. If your child demonstrates uncertainty on his face and you give him a reassuring look, they will recognize the expression and perceive that everything is okay.

At this stage, children begin to seek affection. You might find your baby reaching out to you, starting to snuggle with you, and being proactive toward being held and hugged.

This is also a time when curiosity is piqued. As babies move around, they become more aware of their environment and start to explore it. Seeing and hearing what is going on around them in their world creates a sense of wonderment. Even if your child is not yet creeping independently, they may still want to explore things, whether with you or on their own. Pay attention to the level of curiosity your child is demonstrating.

Finally, babies not only notice the presence of familiar objects but also if they disappear. This is called *object permanence*. If you remove a toy that is near your child, he will recognize that it is gone and look for it. If something drops from the tray in their high chair—a spoon or morsel of food—they will notice that it is missing and look around for it. Playing peekaboo now becomes a fun game.

LEVEL 4: EIGHT TO TWELVE MONTHS

Now that we've covered the lower parts of the brain, you can see how these create a foundation. If you were going to build a house, you know that first a foundation must be laid. The medulla, pons, and midbrain—the brain stem—are critical foundation points in brain development. What comes next is the growth of the cortex. Developmentally, we've divided the cortex stage into five levels, ranging from eight months to school age.

SEEING AND READING

By twelve months of age, a child's vision should automatically support consistent depth perception. This is the ability to see and determine spatial relationships with things and objects around us, and to see in three dimensions, both close-up and at a distance. Now that the child is walking, keen depth perception is vital for interacting with the environment. An example of this is recognizing and understanding how to step up to or down off a curb—your brain knows automatically how your legs will navigate your way on or off a sidewalk when you cross a street. In an organized brain, both eyes work together through the pons and midbrain to create peripheral vision to convergence and now for depth perception. The brain can begin to judge accurately how much distance or height is needed for all motor and visual tasks. For example, without that organization, it would be hard to recognize the difference in height between the sidewalk and the road.

How do you know if your child is lacking depth perception? Can she walk up and down steps easily? Some children have challenges distinguishing between a step and a line on the floor. Some will frequently trip, bump into things, or hesitate when approaching the threshold of a doorway. Others might have a hard time stacking building blocks or placing an item on a table, catching a ball, running quickly, tying their shoes, and perhaps buttoning their shirt. If your child has strabismus, this will automatically impede the development of depth perception. In fact, dynamic depth perception is unlikely.

HEARING AND UNDERSTANDING

Can your child understand at least ten words and simple combinations of words? Not only hearing the words, but also understanding what each word connects to, like "mommy," "daddy," and "peekaboo." The same goes for understanding basic combinations of words and short phrases like

"Are you hungry?" How about simple instructions or requests? Do they recognize familiar people like grandparents and babysitters? Do they recognize the places you frequently visit, like the doctor's office or the toy store?

During this stage, children start to demonstrate the ability to connect people, places, things, and events with joy—or even displeasure or fear, depending on past experiences.

This is also the stage where children become aware of basic time concepts, such as "wait" or "almost ready" or "be right back." They understand that "wait" means just for a moment and that "I'm getting your food" means that if you pop into the kitchen to bring out a dish, you're coming back in short order.

SENSATION AND TACTILITY

If you put your hand in your purse or your coat pocket, you'll be able to notice the difference between the items you touch or hold. Some are sharp (like keys), others are round and hard (like coins), and some things are long (like a pen) or smooth (like a wallet). At this initial cortical tactile level, you'll also notice that you use different pressure or movement in your hand—three-dimensional positioning (stereo gnostic sense)—when holding each item. This three-dimensional-touch factor is like that of visual depth perception and auditory location. Your brain knows what is being touched and how to automatically adjust your hand around the object and grasp it appropriately.

In your child's world, ability applies to how a toy is grabbed, held, or manipulated, and your child should be able to do this with each hand. Given the child's ability to grasp, if she struggles to automatically correct the three-dimensional positioning in either hand when attempting to grab an object or hold an object when it is placed in her hand, this would indicate disorganization in the tactile pathway.

LOCOMOTION AND MOBILITY

At this stage, babies are more mobile and can creep on their hands and knees. Once they reach a piece of furniture, they will grab hold with their hands and pull themselves up. Many will even cruise/walk a few steps while holding on to the furniture. As steadiness, organization, and confidence build, they begin to control gravity, become more bold, and take more and more steps using their arms for balance, between the furniture, or between Mom and Dad. Added encouragement by a parent or family member helps to motivate the walking as well as the child's desire to reach a toy or a pet. At this point, good solid walking on steady feet is an indication of integrated medulla reflexes and good structural development through the consistent function provided by commando crawling and creeping on hands and knees.

COMMUNICATION AND SPEECH

In language, a well-organized, twelve-month-old child should be speaking at least four individual words or using distinct signs (standard sign language). These aren't words you say that they repeat or imitate, but words that come from the child directly of their own volition. The words/signs don't have to be accurately stated but expressed in a way you can understand them, like "mama" for mom or "dada" for dad. It might not be the entire word or a perfectly crafted sign, but if your child uses it to identify someone or something *on a daily basis*, and you recognize the usage and intent, that would count as meaningful communication. These words/signs will probably be reflecting something your child sees or wants.

SIGN LANGUAGE ACTIVATES THE LANGUAGE PATHWAYS AND PROMOTES LANGUAGE

Babies who use signs have been found to have better overall verbal skills, and by the age of eight years, they have higher IQs.

Studies also show that children with special needs benefit from learning sign language.

The same part of the brain (Broca's area) is activated when speaking as when signing.

Understanding receptive language involves more variation in brain activity, the main difference being that the "hearing" person listens to the spoken language activating their auditory cortex while when "signing" the occipital lobe (visual cortex) is activated.

MANUAL AND WRITING

As they approach their first birthday, children begin to use their opposing thumbs and forefingers in a precise pincer grip in each hand to pick up small objects. This is called *cortical opposition*. At the same time, because of this new cortical ability, children are developing the skill to wrap their hands around a spoon or a fork and begin feeding themselves, as well as hold a cup with handles and drink from it.

EMOTIONAL AND SOCIAL

Emotional and social interactions are starting to emerge. You can play interactive games with your child, like hide-and-seek, and she will respond and play along. This is also the phase when children begin to miss you if you're not around—many become concerned, upset, or even cry.

Imitating behavior also emerges. If you're tossing clothes into the laundry basket, your child will do the same. If you make a sound, she will repeat it.

Asserting position and testing boundaries should also occur at this point. You may tell your child not to touch something, then moments later they defy you. They might even turn and look at you while performing this defiant action to make sure you are watching. This is a real test of boundaries and who decides them—you or the child. It is also a sign of initial independence and cognitive awareness, and children will test you more and more as they attempt to understand the importance and extent of the rules you set for them and where the boundaries are. This is brain organization in action.

Experimenting comes now, too. Your child might pick up an item and take a good look at it—feel it, smell it, shake it, or put it in their mouth. Perhaps they drop it to see what will happen. Is your child investigating or experimenting with the things they come across? Or are they apprehensive? Do you have to show them what to do or how to use the item before they can warm up to something new? Some children don't have that ability to experiment with an object themselves, but they're interested in what happens, so you might have to be the one to say, "Look at this," and demonstrate for them. If children tend to prefer the same toy, movie, or book and shy away from new experiences, it can indicate disorganization in the limbic brain.

Finally, there is the ability to transition from one situation to another. For example, if your child is busy playing with a toy, but you need to run an errand, how easy or difficult is it to get them to stop their activity, help them put on their shoes and coat, and leave the house? Some children are challenged by this transition because they are not comfortable moving from one place or situation to another, even if you positively communicate that it's "time to eat."

It is ideal if your child is comfortable with daily transitions—like going from home to the car, the car to the playground, the playground to the supermarket, and the supermarket to home.

BRAIN LEVEL	CORTEX • 4 8 TO 12 MONTHS	YOUR CHILD'S SCORE
SEEING AND READING	• See in three dimensions, perceiving depth • Begin to have far-point depth perception	
HEARING AND UNDERSTANDING	• Understand at least ten common words and basic couplets • Understand/follow simple requests • Remember simple events and familiar people • Understand basic time concepts, such as "wait" and "in a moment"	
SENSATION AND TACTILITY	• Feel the dynamic tactile relationships in three-dimensional objects	
LOCOMOTION AND MOBILITY	• Independently and consistently walk three meters across the room using the arms for balance	
COMMUNICATION AND SPEECH	• Voluntarily communicate with four meaningful words/signs that are understood by parents	
MANUAL AND WRITING	• Cortically oppose thumb and finger in each hand • Begin feeding self using a utensil • Hold a cup and drink from it	
EMOTIONAL AND SOCIAL LIMBIC BRAIN	• Participate in interactive play • Seek parents, objects when moved out of sight • Start to imitate behavior • Assert position; begin to test boundaries • Experiment with a variety of objects • Transition smoothly from one situation to another	

LEVEL 5: TWELVE TO EIGHTEEN MONTHS

We now move on to the phase when cortical functions become more visible and consistent. These abilities should become well organized within eighteen months.

SEEING AND READING

In this phase, a child recognizes pictures, sees detailed images, and associates a photo with a person or a thing that is meaningful. For example, your child sees a picture of Dad or Grandma, readily recognizes who is in the photo, and gets excited. Or, if there is a picture of a dog in a storybook, your child looks for your dog because they are making that association and that connection. This means that your child can perceive pictures as abstract representations of actual objects.

HEARING AND UNDERSTANDING

By now, a child can usually understand at least fifty words as well as phrases and simple sentences. This includes being able to comprehend and respond to a two-step request like, "Pick up your cup and give it to me." Can your child do that? Can they look for the cup and deliver it to you? That's a two-step request in action.

This is also the stage when children have a sense of what a typical day entails: the basic routines and the daily timing of events. For example, at bedtime, you have a nice routine in place. You help your child change into pajamas, put him to bed, read a story, turn out the lights, give a good-night kiss, and close the bedroom door. But what if you have a night where you're exhausted or have another responsibility that evening, and you need to pass on story time? You tuck your child into his bed, kiss him good night, and walk out of the room. And what happens? He starts protesting, right? That bedtime story is part of the overall nightly routine, and because you've changed the routine, he doesn't let you off the hook. This "knowing" about what comes next and understanding the daily routine is part of your child's development. In fact, he is beginning to learn many of the routines that are part of his day, such as eating breakfast, getting changed and dressed, bathing, car rides, and so on.

SENSATION AND TACTILITY

Tactile ability comes to the forefront now. Your child will be able to recognize familiar items and toys by touch. They can put their hand in the toy box and know what they're looking for, whether it's a ball or a toy car. They can feel their way among the various items in the toy box and distinguish between them without looking.

LOCOMOTION AND MOBILITY

At this point, a child can stand up in the middle of the floor without needing a piece of furniture or their arms for balance. Walking should be the primary way in which the child gets around now, and they should be able to do so in an unrestricted and balanced manner without the knees bent, the feet turning in, on their toes, or with a disorganized, awkward gait.

COMMUNICATION AND SPEECH

By the time they reach eighteen months old, children should be starting to say twenty meaningful words and at least three meaningful couplets (combining two words). In this case, "meaningful" means voluntary and relevant to the moment. This does not mean repeating something picked up from another person or the TV. These should be words that your child is using to communicate directly with you, like "I want," "play ball," or our favorite, "What's that?"

If you have a nonverbal child who uses sign language to communicate in a similarly meaningful way, this will also count.

MANUAL AND WRITING

Children can use their thumbs and forefingers—cortical opposition—to pick up items in each hand simultaneously. They can also use both hands to grasp objects, like building blocks, and hold one block in the left hand while stacking the second block with the right hand. This skill is also apparent in the child who is starting to dress and undress himself, like when taking off shoes, socks, or a hat using both hands together. This entails a more sophisticated bilateral use of cortical opposition to accomplish tasks.

EMOTIONAL AND SOCIAL

In the emotional and social areas, children should be making meaningful eye contact while communicating. Limbic system injuries or visual challenges make it difficult to communicate using eye contact when interacting with other people. Typical eye contact entails sustaining that contact for a reasonable period within a conversation to show acknowledgment and interest (as opposed to either avoiding eye contact altogether or staring at someone directly for a prolonged amount of time). Does your child come into a room, look at you, and then talk? Or do they enter the room talking but without making eye contact with you?

Is your child happy when they should be happy and sad when they should be sad? You should notice your child expressing a good range of appropriate emotions and having some initial ability to self-regulate. This might be displayed, for example, through the excitement your child demonstrates when Daddy comes home from work. On the other hand, an overly emotional reaction would be exhibiting too much hugging or clinging, or else sustaining exuberance for too long a time. The same would apply when showing anger and frustration—if there's too much anger displayed leading to extended or frequent tantrums or lack of control, there could be a problem. By and large, children in this age range should demonstrate a good variety of healthy emotions (anger, excitement, anticipation, sadness, disappointment, jealousy) expressed appropriately and in balance, with moderate self-control.

BRAIN LEVEL	CORTEX • 5 12 TO 18 MONTHS	YOUR CHILD'S SCORE
SEEING AND READING	• Perceive pictures as abstract representations of concrete objects	
HEARING AND UNDERSTANDING	• Understand at least 50 words, as well as phrases and simple sentences • Understand/follow a simple two-step request • Understand the time relationships of a typical day	
SENSATION AND TACTILITY	• Locate a favorite toy by feel with each hand, without looking	
LOCOMOTION AND MOBILITY	• Stand up in the middle of the floor independently and walk three meters, without using arms for balance • Walk as a means of transportation in an unrestricted and coordinated cross pattern	
COMMUNICATION AND SPEECH	• Voluntarily communicate with 20 meaningful single words/signs • Voluntarily communicate with at least three meaningful couplets using words/signs	
MANUAL AND WRITING	• Use both hands together, cortically opposing the thumb and finger • Build structures using blocks • Begin basic dressing and undressing— taking off socks/shoes	
EMOTIONAL AND SOCIAL LIMBIC BRAIN	• Make good eye contact while communicating, including joint attention • Express wide range of emotions appropriately • Play alongside other children (parallel play) with adult support • Engage in purposeful activities	

How does your child connect with other children? If in a supervised environment, like the playground, when your child sees other children can they sit nearby and play along with them? Do they learn from watching others play and begin to imitate what other children are doing? Parallel play—independently playing alongside other children—is a new stage that demonstrates awareness of how other children do things. We adults do this all the time by watching others in our field of interest and copying what we view as important.

The same applies to how your child engages in purposeful activities, rather than wandering around or throwing toys, when you are in the same room. Pay attention to what your child is doing, how engaged or disengaged he is in that activity, and how engaged he is with you if you're nearby. Also, observe how your child plays with his toys.

LEVEL 6: EIGHTEEN TO THIRTY-SIX MONTHS

SEEING AND READING

By thirty-six months, if given ample opportunity, children can recognize and identify numbers from one to ten and most, if not all, letters of the alphabet. They can see a number or letter and know it's a *2, 3, a,* or *b*. Some children might confuse a *b* with a *d*, so make note if that happens consistently.

Children with verbal challenges who can point to things may be able to readily identify numbers or letters they see in a book or on a license plate. If they know and can point to or verbally identify all the letters and basic numbers you're asking them about, they're proficient.

HEARING AND UNDERSTANDING

When it comes to hearing and understanding language, by now, children should be able to comprehend thousands of words along with simple paragraphs. If you are reading a book aloud, they will pay attention to stories that have pictures, paragraphs, and a basic theme. You can begin to reason with children at this level. They can also follow basic and related three-step requests without you pointing out or repeating the request when they get stuck. An example: "Please get your shoes and teddy bear and meet me by the front door." That's a three-step instruction in which the child hears, understands, and follows through on all the actions.

Children should also understand the basic time concepts of *yesterday, today,* and *tomorrow*. You should be able to talk to your child about something you did together the day before—"Did you have fun at the park yesterday?"—as well as whatever is happening today and planned for tomorrow. That would include anticipation of what will happen later today, as in, "After lunch, let's play a game." Children are usually adept at reminding you of something you promised to do together later in the day or the next day.

An understanding of spatial concepts like *underneath, on top of,* and *around* also comes into play. So if you say, "Please put your cup on the table," your child will understand what to do.

SENSATION AND TACTILITY

At this stage, children can feel and identify objects by their physical characteristics—like hard, soft, round, and flat—with each hand. If you ask your child to give you the soft one, the round one, or the long one, they can place their hand in the toy box (using their hands and not their eyes) and distinguish between two items and give it to you. That is excellent.

LOCOMOTION AND MOBILITY

Children can now "escape" gravity, land in a coordinated way, and run independently. To achieve this level, the running should be in a coordinated, airborne cross-pattern manner—heel to toe—for at least ten meters nonstop. They can easily balance and hop on two feet or either foot a few times without falling.

COMMUNICATION AND SPEECH

Children can now put together meaningful, organized sentences on a daily basis. These sentences will increase from three to four words up to five to six words and be spoken consistently. They can also take those sentences and create a little story by stringing together at least three short sentences without any prompting (and similar to the three-step request). An example: "Mommy, I heard a noise, and I looked out the window, and a tree fell down." If something occurs, your child can tell you about it in the order of events.

Language is very clear and virtually nonstop at this stage. Not only can you understand what your child is saying, but others can, too. There might be a word here or there that lacks a bit of clarity, but overall you should be able to understand them.

MANUAL AND WRITING

By now, children are using both of their hands together, freely, for a variety of different skills that are slightly more sophisticated—turning on a faucet, opening a door, screwing and unscrewing a basic jar—and performing these actions as quickly and easily as their peers.

They are also becoming more adept at dressing and undressing, using their dominant hand during the task. This includes buttoning and unbuttoning big buttons, unzipping a jacket, pulling up pants, and taking off and putting on a shirt.

Children can pour liquid into a cup using two hands—one to hold the cup and the other to pour. Depth perception is in play here, as well.

EMOTIONAL AND SOCIAL

In the emotional and social areas, children now recognize the link between behavior and consequences, because they've tested enough boundaries at this stage. Life experiences, parents, and caregivers have taught them what is and isn't okay, and they can distinguish between the two and begin to think for a moment, pausing before they act. If they've been told not to climb up on the sofa and onto the coffee table and jump on the floor, they now know what will happen if they do this activity. Once the rules have been consistently applied, they should understand that there will be consequences. Children will then begin to consider their actions and the possible outcomes before they undertake them.

If children continue to repeat the same inappropriate behavior, it could mean the boundaries aren't clear to them and/or that they have some neurological disorganization.

Sharing is another concept that children learn and apply. It's the beginning of commerce—making an agreement and, at the same time, exhibiting altruistic behavior. In a supervised environment, can your child share a toy with a playmate of her own volition? Would she share something with a friend if you asked her to do so? Would she object if another child took something from her without asking? Most children are willing to share at this stage. They are even aware of how others share with them and share items of equal value, such as a truck with a ball. Sharing happens when the prefrontal cortex starts to come "online." Adults help navigate the virtues of sharing so that the give-and-take nature inherent in the act of sharing begins to make sense for a child.

This is also the stage when children participate in role-playing and fantasy games to practice being an adult. They will play with cars, trucks, and animals, creating different scenarios. You might see your child trying to walk around the house wearing your shoes, pretending to be a favorite character from a movie, or carrying a baby doll or a sword and pretending to be a doctor or construction worker. Your child will do this alone or with a sibling or friend. Together, they create mini scenarios around these characters and act them out. This activity is a way to express emotions (adult concept formation).

Developing a natural and *spontaneous* interest in being helpful to others is a delightful milestone to see your child reach. They may put their finished juice box in the trash, help you sort the laundry, or comfort

BRAIN LEVEL	CORTEX • 6 18 TO 36 MONTHS	YOUR CHILD'S SCORE
SEEING AND READING	• Recognize and identify numerals • Recognize and identify letters of the alphabet	
HEARING AND UNDERSTANDING	• Understand thousands of words and simple paragraphs • Understand/follow a basic three-step request • Understand basic time concepts, such as yesterday, today, and tomorrow • Understand basic spatial concepts, such as underneath, on top of, and around	
SENSATION AND TACTILITY	• Feel and identify an object by its physical characteristics (hard, soft, round, flat) with each hand	
LOCOMOTION AND MOBILITY	• Independently run ten meters nonstop • Independently run in an unrestricted and coordinated cross pattern • Hop in place on one foot	
COMMUNICATION AND SPEECH	• Voluntarily put a meaningful, organized sentence together • Voluntarily tell a meaningful, organized short story • Speak as clearly as peers	
MANUAL AND WRITING	• Use hands for sophisticated skills (button, zip, screw) as quickly and easily as peers • Dress and undress using one hand in a lead role • Pour liquid using one hand in a lead role	
EMOTIONAL AND SOCIAL LIMBIC BRAIN	• Recognize link between behaviors and consequences • Share toys and play with others (supervised) • Engage in fantasy games and role-playing to express emotion and concept formation • Spontaneously help others • Refer to self using "me" or "I" • Feel and display remorse and pride	

a baby sibling who is crying. This isn't just imitating behavior observed at home, it is understanding and applying it unselfishly, or being part of an activity you engage in, like clearing the dinner table or putting away groceries.

In language, if your child is verbal, you will find they will begin to refer to themselves in the first person as "me" or "I," rather than by their name or in the third person. This is a huge milestone in prefrontal lobe organization/development. They are now beginning to notice that they are unique and may spend time looking in the mirror and wondering, Who am I and how do I fit in?

With this individualization underway, children begin to feel and display remorse and pride. They identify as their own person, one who is different from you. If they do something positive, they are excited by it and want to share it with you. For example, you can see the sense of accomplishment and pride on their face and they may look to you or bring you a drawing or something they have created.

The same goes for remorse. If they do something "wrong," they now feel sorry about it. This process occurs because the prefrontal cortex is becoming more organized. So if your child accidentally knocks a vase off a table and it breaks, or he hurts another child, he should feel sorry about it and want to reconcile with you. If you notice that your child is feeling remorse, this is neurologically excellent.

MOVING THROUGH THE LEVELS

At this point in the process, you may find that you're approaching the apex of your child's current developmental level. If this is the case, and if you wish, you can proceed to the end of this chapter to learn how to put this information all together.

If you have other children in your family, moving forward into levels seven and eight will give you more information about how they are doing with their development.

LEVEL 7: THIRTY-SIX TO SEVENTY-TWO MONTHS

This level covers the period from ages three to six. This is the time period, neurologically, when many high-level abilities begin to solidify.

SEEING AND READING

From a visual standpoint, reading now comes into play. If your child has been taught to read, he can recognize fifty words and master these words in different ways, such as identifying them in couplets or phrases when you're reading a book together or else matching a word and couplets to a picture.

HEARING AND UNDERSTANDING

As you read to or with your child, as he matures, so do the books you choose. The books will gradually contain more words so that, eventually, words predominate and pictures are limited to the beginnings of chapters. The more mature the reader becomes, the more stories will have a clear theme with a beginning, middle, and end. As children age from three to six, they become more adept at listening to and comprehending a story with more paragraphs and an intricate plot. The same goes for watching a movie. They can follow the plot and understand (and be curious about) the what, where, why, when, and how. More considerable attention to detail is now needed. Five- to six-year-olds can follow chapter books and recall the details of one chapter as they get to the next, even if there is a short lapse in time.

Children can also follow a four-step request. At bedtime, they should be able to comply with the request to undress, put on pajamas, brush their teeth, and choose a book for a bedtime story.

Games become an integral part of play now, whether it is a simple board game, cards, tag, or any other type of indoor or outdoor game. Children should be able to understand the rules of the game, the basic moves, and game etiquette like patiently waiting their turn. They should also be able to read the numbers on the spinner or dice.

When it comes to numbers, simple math concepts should be understood at this time. *How many people are in our family? How many plates do we put on the table for dinner? If Grandma and Grandpa visit, how many more people will be at the dinner table?* This knowledge sets the foundation for understanding basic arithmetic once school starts.

Finally, and importantly, can your child remain safely left alone for short periods of time? If you leave the room temporarily to bring up the laundry or go to the bathroom, does your child know not to turn on the stove or light matches? To look both ways crossing the street? Do they know where not to go in the garage and what tools are sharp or dangerous? Are they aware enough to warn other siblings not to go into dangerous areas? If they get lost in a store, can they seek help?

SENSATION AND TACTILITY

If you give your child a coin, they should be able to feel both sides and distinguish heads from tails with each hand without looking. Many five- and six-year-olds can do this, so with a little practice, they will be able to tell the difference and do so with each hand.

LOCOMOTION AND MOBILITY

Once a child can hop on one foot, the next ability is hopping all the way across the room on one foot. Then hopping all the way back on the other foot at a distance of about five meters (about five yards).

COMMUNICATION AND SPEECH

At this time, language becomes more sophisticated, and children consistently speak in paragraphs. A three- to four-year-old can tell a story consisting of three or four sentences, while a six-year-old will talk much longer and in greater detail. Children are sequentially expressing ideas and information consistently about an event, a story, or a film. Can your child watch a movie, comprehend the story, and then tell you about it in an organized way so that you understand what it is about?

While many children can talk up a storm during this time, some might only be able to talk about a story they have created, rather than describe something that has happened to them in a way that makes sense to another person. Your child needs to be independent in her ability to communicate and express herself.

MANUAL AND WRITING

When drawing, your child should demonstrate the ability to create people with distinct body parts, such as a face, arms, and legs. Hands might also be drawn but not necessarily fingers. Small details might make their way into the drawing, like eyeglasses or a beard. In early drawings, children can draw a head, along with a face with eyes, nose, and a mouth. The arms and legs are attached to the head. As they progress, children begin to separate the body from the head and there may be an additional detail, like hair. The older the child, the more features will be added.

The following are two examples of a typical drawing by a four-year-old and a six-year-old.

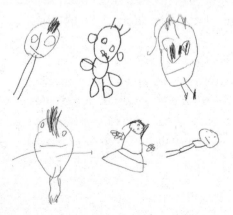

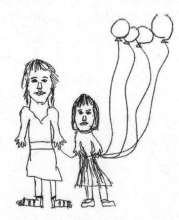

When it comes to writing, this is more complex, as children have to take information and words that are in their brain and move that through the hand onto a page. They can now write about ten words and five couplets that are readable. Spelling might not be perfect, but it is basic and understandable.

EMOTIONAL AND SOCIAL

At this stage, children can start to see the "big picture." They are developing the ability to work together with others and solve problems. If something is wrong, they will figure out a way to fix it and to work cooperatively with the family. If you're leaving the house for the day, your child might realize he forgot his backpack and then go to his room to retrieve it. Or he might see a younger sibling struggling to reach a toy on a shelf and help by reaching up and grabbing that toy for his sister.

It is also a time for engaging in a team or group setting and following the rules of the group. Can she be with more than one person at a time? If so, how many? How old are the other children in that group?

By now, children not only understand the link between behavior and consequences, but they also know how to modify their behavior over the period of the day to achieve a positive outcome and/or to avoid an adverse one. They begin to catch themselves behaving in ways they shouldn't—like being disruptive, talking too loudly, or playing too rough—and adjust their actions accordingly. They understand what parents expect of them, as well as the boundaries set for them. They also know that there could be a negative outcome when they don't comply.

The understanding of emotions and their causes also comes into play now. Children begin to recognize how they are feeling and develop insight into *why* they may feel sad or upset. They can identify what occurred to trigger that emotion and can express it to their parents. They can also reflect on similar circumstances and see how things eventually changed or improved.

BRAIN LEVEL	CORTEX • 7 36 TO 72 MONTHS	YOUR CHILD'S SCORE
SEEING AND READING	• Read at least 50 single words and simple phrases	
HEARING AND UNDERSTANDING	• Understand complex paragraphs and stories • Follow a common four-step request • Understand/follow basic concepts in organized games • Understand simple mathematical concepts • Safely remain alone for short periods	
SENSATION AND TACTILITY	• Feel the difference between sophisticated and similar objects, e.g. can determine the difference between two sides of a coin, with each hand	
LOCOMOTION AND MOBILITY	• Independently and bilaterally hop across a room five meters nonstop	
COMMUNICATION AND SPEECH	• Voluntarily use organized paragraphs to express ideas • Sequentially express information, as in a short story, event, or movie	
MANUAL AND WRITING	• Draw people with distinct body parts • Voluntarily write ten words • Voluntarily write five couplets • Write clearly	
EMOTIONAL AND SOCIAL LIMBIC BRAIN	• Work with others, and seek opportunities to solve problems for the family • Engage in a team or group setting and follow the rules of the group • Modify behavior to achieve a positive outcome and/or avoid a negative outcome • Begin to gain insight into possible causes of emotions	

LEVEL 8: CHRONOLOGICAL AGE LEVEL (AGE SIX AND ABOVE)

By the age of six, most children have started school and should be performing at a chronological age level. This is also the point at which they will demonstrate uniform hemispheric dominance.

In early development, children switch back and forth, moving from one dominant eye to the other, one dominant ear to the other. Eventually, they integrate the process, which makes it possible to become fully lateralized. As you may recall, there are two sides of the brain—the right and the left hemispheres. The right hemisphere runs the left side of the body; the left hemisphere controls the right side of the body. One side should be the leader consistently. So if your left brain is the leader, you're going to be right-handed, right-footed, right-eyed, and right-eared. If you're switching back and forth, you might be right-eyed, but sometimes left-eyed, or sometimes using your right hand and sometimes using your left hand. You might hop on your right foot but kick a soccer ball with the left foot. You might be thoroughly mixed up in your dominance, and if that's the case, that crossover can also cause reversing of letters, or you flip hemispheres while reading, which results in seeing the left and right sides of a page but missing what's in the middle. To read well, to retrieve information well, you need to have a consistent hemispheric dominance. You probably weren't aware of this, but now that you are, you can observe your child to better understand how the last part of the cerebrum is organized.

In measuring the school-age child, you will factor in the chronological age and will do so in months, not years. For example, if your child is ten, they would be one hundred and twenty months. If academically and developmentally they are performing at age level with no extra help or guidance from you or teachers (and essentially independent with no adaptions to the environment), that would be noted as one hundred twenty months as well. However, if they perform at the level of an eight-year-old, that would be ninety-six months, and that would be noted as the basic age.

As you go through each of the following seven brain functions, consider what your child is learning at school and how proficiently he is performing. If you notice a shift in the child's hemisphere dominance, make a note of that, too.

SEEING AND READING

Children can read, both with content comprehension and with speed, as well as their peers at grade level.

HEARING AND UNDERSTANDING

The hearing is functioning well, and children can understand sophisticated life concepts and relationships on par with their peers. How are they keeping up with their peers academically? Are they independent or do they need extra time and support to do their work?

SENSATION AND TACTILITY

Observe which hand your child is using for various activities to see which is dominant and whether they are using that hand proficiently. They should demonstrate uniform hemispheric dominance at this time.

LOCOMOTION AND MOBILITY

Your child should be able to learn new physical skills and become proficient in new physical challenges that match those of peers. If you enroll your child in sports—like a tennis class—observe how well they are learning and if their skills are evolving as well as the other children on their team or in their group.

Children at this level should be able to swim, ride a bicycle without training wheels, and learn new physical skills akin to their peers. If they do not, compare their coordination skills with other children in their age group.

COMMUNICATION AND SPEECH

How well is your child speaking? They should be able to voluntarily talk and express ideas as well as their peers in vocabulary, content, tonality, and clarity.

MANUAL AND WRITING

At this level, children can write organized sentences and paragraphs. The writing is legible, and thoughts and ideas are expressed clearly on paper in a spontaneous manner.

EMOTIONAL AND SOCIAL

As children mature, they become more adept at considering the needs and emotions of others at their age level. They are also motivated to meet both their own needs and the needs of others.

This is also a time for engaging in group activities with peers and developing meaningful and appropriate relationships. They should be particularly comfortable among their peers.

Children can defer gratification, so when things don't happen as planned or as anticipated, they can roll with it or get over the natural disappointment or frustration more quickly than they used to. They also know that they can make another plan for another time and have something to look forward to.

This is also a time for developing meaningful, mutually beneficial friendships as well as providing for their own needs and those of others. If your child invites a friend over to play and gets hungry, they won't just come to you for a snack for themselves, but also consider whether the friend might like one, too.

BRAIN LEVEL	CORTEX • 8 CHRONOLOGICAL AGE	YOUR CHILD'S SCORE
SEEING AND READING	• Read in content and speed as well as peers • Demonstrate uniform hemispheric dominance	
HEARING AND UNDERSTANDING	• Understand sophisticated life concepts and relationships as well as peers • Demonstrate uniform hemispheric dominance	
SENSATION AND TACTILITY	• Demonstrate uniform hemispheric dominance	
LOCOMOTION AND MOBILITY	• Become proficient in new physical challenges as quickly as peers • Learn new physical skills as quickly as peers • Demonstrate uniform hemispheric dominance	
COMMUNICATION AND SPEECH	• Voluntarily speak and express ideas as well as peers	
MANUAL AND WRITING	• Write organized sentences • Write organized paragraphs • Write thoughts spontaneously and voluntarily as well as peers • Write clearly • Demonstrate uniform hemispheric dominance	
EMOTIONAL AND SOCIAL LIMBIC BRAIN	• Consider thoughts, needs, and emotions of others • Engage in group activities with peers independently • Defer gratification • Develop meaningful and appropriate relationships • Self-motivated to meet own needs and others' needs	

PUTTING IT ALL TOGETHER

You've gone through the process of evaluating your child's current brain function. Now you're ready to take all your information—all the As, NAs, PAs, and NYAs you marked on the charts. If you've been making these notes elsewhere, transfer this information to the charts.

To begin, review your responses in the "Your Child's Score" boxes at each level. If a box has multiple bullet points, look at how you responded to each bullet and then calculate an *average* for that section. Consider the example below.

SEEING AND READING	• See and distinguish details from three meters • See changes in facial expression • Bring eyes together and converge vision on an object	*NA* *A* *NA* (*NA*)

Since there are two NAs together with an A, the score would be NA (circled). In fact, any box that has NA bullet points combined with A bullet points should automatically get an overall score of NA. If you have a box with bullet points with a variety of PA, NA, and NYA scores, make the box score an overall PA.

For example:

Three NAs and two PAs = PA
Four NAs and one PA = PA
Two As, two NAs, and two PAs = NA

Do this for every box you completed, leaving each box containing *one* assessment score. Use your best judgment as to your child's overall achievement within each box.

Following are two charts. The first one is a simple grid you can use to help summarize the overall neurological function of your child. The second chart is an example of a the completed chart of a child we saw in the clinic. The grayed-out areas to the right are for those skills this child hasn't yet achieved or isn't chronologically mature enough to achieve.

You can draw a vertical line separating out the areas/columns where your child displays no further abilities. In many cases, this dividing line is uneven. This is typical for a hurt child.

THE FAMILY HOPE CENTER
INTEGRATIVE AND DEVELOPMENTAL PROGRESSION CHART

BRAIN LEVEL	MEDULLA OBLONGATA • 1	PONS • 2	MIDBRAIN • 3	CORTEX • 4	CORTEX • 5	CORTEX • 6	CORTEX • 7	CORTEX • 8
DEVELOPMENTAL PERIOD	BIRTH TO 0.5 MONTHS	0.5 MONTHS TO 2 MONTHS	2 TO 8 MONTHS	8 TO 12 MONTHS	12 TO 18 MONTHS	18 TO 36 MONTHS	36 TO 72 MONTHS	CHRON. AGE LEVEL
SEEING AND READING								
HEARING AND UNDERSTANDING								
SENSATION AND TACTILITY								
LOCOMOTION AND MOBILITY								
COMMUNICATION AND SPEECH								
MANUAL AND WRITING								
EMOTIONAL AND SOCIAL — LIMBIC BRAIN								

Now that you have done a deep dive into your child's brain, there are three major pieces of information we must extract from the chart to "see" the child and eventually know where to begin healing their brain.

THE FAMILY HOPE CENTER
INTEGRATIVE AND DEVELOPMENTAL PROGRESSION CHART

NAME: *Your Child's Evaluation*   DATE OF BIRTH: *DOB*   TODAY'S DATE: *Today*

<table>
<tr><td rowspan="2">BRAIN FUNCTION</td><td></td><td>BRAIN LEVEL</td><td>MEDULLA OBLONGATA • 1</td><td>PONS • 2</td><td>MIDBRAIN • 3</td></tr>
<tr><td></td><td>DEVELOPMENTAL PERIOD</td><td>BIRTH TO 0.5 MONTHS</td><td>0.5 MONTHS TO 2 MONTHS</td><td>2 TO 8 MONTHS</td></tr>
<tr><td rowspan="3">SENSORY</td><td>SEEING AND READING</td><td>NA</td><td>NA</td><td>NA</td></tr>
<tr><td>HEARING AND UNDERSTANDING</td><td>PA</td><td>NYA</td><td>PA</td></tr>
<tr><td>SENSATION AND TACTILITY</td><td>NA</td><td>NA</td><td>NA</td></tr>
<tr><td rowspan="3">MOTOR</td><td>LOCOMOTION AND MOBILITY</td><td>A</td><td>NA</td><td>NA</td></tr>
<tr><td>COMMUNICATION AND SPEECH</td><td>A</td><td>A</td><td>NA</td></tr>
<tr><td>MANUAL AND WRITING</td><td>NA</td><td>A</td><td>A</td></tr>
<tr><td>SOCIAL</td><td>EMOTIONAL AND SOCIAL — LIMBIC BRAIN</td><td>NA</td><td>A</td><td>NA</td></tr>
</table>

CHRONOLOGICAL AGE: _36_   INITIAL CHRONOLOGICAL AGE: _____

NEUROLOGICAL AGE: _11.52_   INITIAL NEUROLOGICAL AGE: _____

CORTEX • 4	CORTEX • 5	CORTEX • 6	CORTEX • 7	CORTEX • 8
8 TO 12 MONTHS	12 TO 18 MONTHS	18 TO 36 MONTHS	36 TO 72 MONTHS	CHRONOLOGICAL AGE LEVEL
PA	A			
NA	PA			
A				
A	NA			
A				
PA				
PA				

We need to know:

- the extent of the injury,
- the areas of the brain affected, and
- the degree of the injury.

You've achieved the amazing task of understanding the brain areas and pathways of the chart. Congratulate yourself and pause. Take a deep breath. Remember that data is empowering, though it can at first feel completely overwhelming. You're ready to address the extent and areas of the brain that are compromised.

What the NAs, PAs, and NYAs say are only as important as what you do with them. Once we establish this, our next step is to create a plan based on this information that will help your child progress beyond his or her current neurology. Here is where the healing really begins.

To determine the "extent of the injury," simply look at the seven brain functions (Seeing/Reading, Hearing/Understanding, Sensation/Tactile, Locomotion/Mobility, Communication/Speech, Manual/Writing, and Emotional/Social) and determine if any of these pathways are not functioning perfectly. You can see this if any of the boxes along these pathways have an NYA, PA, or NA.

DECIPHERING THE EXTENT OF NEUROLOGICAL FUNCTION	
Centralized	One function compromised
Relatively Centralized	Two to three functions compromised
Relatively Extensive	Four to five functions compromised
Extensive	Six to seven functions compromised

Therefore, the child's injury depicted in the table on pages 142 and 143 is extensive (all seven functions have been compromised).

DETERMINING WHERE BRAIN INJURY IS LOCATED

You can now pinpoint the part (or parts) of the brain in which the injury/ disorganization is located.

Look back at your child's chart, starting with levels one, two, and three. These levels cover the medulla oblongata, the pons, and the midbrain. Levels four through eight cover the cortex.

Are there any NA, PA, or NYA scores noted in these brain areas? Let's look at the sample chart again:

	MEDULLA OBLONGATA 1	PONS 2	MIDBRAIN 3	CORTEX 4	CORTEX 5	CORTEX 6	CORTEX 7	CORTEX 8
SEEING/READING	NA	NA	NA	PA				
HEARING/ UNDERSTANDING	PA	NYA	PA	NA	PA			
SENSATION/ TACTILITY	NA	NA	NA					
LOCOMOTION/ MOBILITY		NA	NA		NA			
COMMUNICATION/ SPEECH			NA					
MANUAL/WRITING	NA			PA				
EMOTIONAL/ SOCIAL	NA		NA	PA				

Notice (looking at the vertical columns) there are NAs and PAs in the medulla (five noted), in the pons (four noted), and the midbrain (six noted). There are signs of injury in the cortex as well. Further, looking horizontally, the Emotional and Social domain draws attention to the function of the limbic brain, and you can see that there are three places in which there are injuries (noted in level one, three, and four).

This means the child has injury in their brain stem, limbic system, and cortex.

The final piece, which is a bit complicated, is to the calculate the degree of injury—that is, to determine the overall neurological age and compare this to the child's chronological age. This gives a parent the percentage of a child's function according to their age. For instance, in the chart above, the child's neurological age, or NA (11.52 months), would be divided by their chronological age, or CA (36 months), giving them a degree of function of 32 percent. We go into this detail in our online training course and also individually when we see a child in the clinic. Our constant endeavor going forward is to "catch up" the NA (neurological age) to the CA (chronological age).

COMING TO TERMS WITH YOUR CHILD'S RESULTS

If you're stunned and unsettled by the extent of compromised areas of the brain, please pause and remember that this is not the end—*it is the beginning*. You may have thought your child was struggling, and even if the neurological picture is what you thought it would be, now that this is on paper in front of you, it can be upsetting and difficult to process.

Perhaps your child is eight, ten, or twelve years old, and now, thinking back over the course of their life, you realize that they plateaued at three or four years old. That could be equally unsettling, due to the sudden awareness that your child's development was not progressing as it should have over the last few years.

This is a baseline measurement of what your child *can do at this moment*. So if you're feeling upset or worried, know that things can get better. You must understand where you are right now to determine where you're going and how to get there. The next chapter begins the journey into the plan.

FAMILY SUCCESS STORY

Our seven-year-old daughter had learning and socializing difficulties during first grade (of elementary school).

Before the program, she displayed many physical symptoms, including abdominal pain and constipation, headache, trouble sleeping, and excessive sweating in her hands and feet. She had difficulty concentrating; cried when she didn't get her way or was unable to explain her feelings; exhibited compulsive behaviors with food, mood swings, sensitivity to sounds; had difficulty making friends or sharing; and suffered low esteem.

A psychologist evaluated our daughter and thought she had a normal IQ, she demonstrated challenging negative behaviors, and needed therapeutic support aimed at restructuring thoughts of anxiety. Before starting the Family Hope Center's program, a psychiatrist evaluated our daughter and confirmed that she had anxiety but recommended that she be medicated.

My husband and I decided to attend the FHC parent training conference in Philadelphia to help our daughter. We found out that her neurological age was five years old and that the gap was caused by her food intolerance (to gluten, sugar, milk, GMOs). We implemented the FHC program, and after six months our daughter reached the level of her peers. We decided to continue the program. Seven months later, her neurological age increased by almost a year. By the end of eighteen months, when our daughter was eight and a half, her neurological age had reached eight as well. She is now a leader, an excellent student, and a sports lover.

Thanks to the Family Hope Center program, she is healthy, successful, and happy.

—*Erika's mom*

NEURO-PARENTING POINTS

- To help heal your child's brain, it is vital to measure developmental abilities and current levels of proficiency.
- Your child has a chronological age and a neurological age. You can measure and assess your child's neurological function by using the Integrative and Developmental Chart (IDPC).
- The IDPC outlines the neurotypical benchmarks for sensory, motor, emotional, and social skills covering seven areas of brain function. Each of these seven areas will be measured over eight developmental levels from birth through six years of age and beyond.
- When assessing your child's proficiency in any of these seven levels of brain function, you will note them as follows:

A	Achieved (Always)
NA	Nearly Achieved (Most of the time)
PA	Partially Achieved (Sometimes)
NYA	Not Yet Achieved (Little to not at all yet)

- Once you have completed your child's assessment using the chart, you can understand your child's neurological situation. Having that baseline measurement of your child's current abilities allows you to create an appropriate plan to help your child progress beyond his current neurology.

CHAPTER 6

BACK TO THE FUTURE: HOW SENSORY STIMULATION AND BASIC MOVEMENT CAN DEVELOP AND IMPROVE BRAIN FUNCTION

he first five chapters have led you to this point in the journey—the place where you can start to develop and heal the brain. In this chapter, we'll explain the principles for promoting neurological growth, and we'll demonstrate how these concepts can be put into a practical approach for your child.

While we hope you've become a more informed neuro-parent and have gained valuable insight into what's happening with your child's brain, we also recognize you're eager to move forward. Since every child is unique and requires an approach tailored specifically to their needs and goals, we realize this book, while informative, can only outline the fundamental principles that apply to most children with special needs, from very mild learning and language concerns, to a child who needs 100 percent of our attention every day.

Moreover, these are concepts and exercises you can wholeheartedly employ with your child today—concepts and exercises with the methods and means that begin the process of reorganizing the brain to help your child better develop. These fundamental and consistent steps can pave the way to improved function.

It's also important to note that this chapter presents a big-picture view of neurodevelopment and neurostimulation (we go into greater detail during our thorough parent training conferences and individual sessions with families).

Nonetheless, if you grasp these principles, you win—and so does your child. As we emphasized early on, as a parent, you're fully equipped with the intention, attention, and consistency to create the change your child needs and deserves.

Efficient and organized sensory competence always precedes any organized motor output. If you're running a software program on your computer and you encounter glitches or it crashes, the solution is to go back and upgrade the software—the effective output is determined by the written software. If you wanted to learn how to ride a bicycle, you would first have to *see* it, *hear* the instructions, and *feel* what it's like to sit on the bicycle, steer it, and work the pedals before you can give it an independent try. The sensory awareness of what it takes to be competent comes before the successful, coordinated physical action. If any motor output is impaired in some way, you must examine the sensory pathway to discover which circuits are disorganized or incomplete and then spend 65 percent of your efforts working to develop them. This development is then reinforced through movement.

When developing the brain, you can't attempt to gain ability if you lack the necessary neurological tools. Otherwise, you wind up managing and adjusting the environment of the child and drifting away from the central issue. Our approach is to identify the current level of function and develop it, naturally progressing to the next level. The beauty and simplicity of the brain is that it grows through extensive use and in an organized fashion. Consider this a bottom-up approach to organization.

Whenever there's a breakdown in the development process, you must start from the current level of function.

FREQUENCY. INTENSITY. DURATION.

A concert pianist. An accomplished athlete. An expert stonemason.

What do these people have in common? Proficiency in their abilities.

What does it take to develop and hone these abilities? *Frequency, intensity, and duration.* It takes all three to effect change and growth.

Frequency = How often?
Intensity = How intense?
Duration = How long?

This strategy applies when helping your child. We've already established that the brain grows physically with stimulation—this is the principle of neuroplasticity, which is the ability of the brain to adapt and change in response to stimulation by making new connections and laying down new pathways.

Over time, this type of effort, not unlike honing an athletic or artistic ability, is a building process that can create positive changes in sensory and motor development. This "bottom-up" rather than "top-down" approach enables the child's brain to make vital connections that foster healing and growth.

Here's an extreme but true example. You discover that your child is functionally blind, and you desperately want to know what it's going to take to get them from a state of blindness to seeing. Seems impossible, right? You've been told that if your child is blind past the age of four, it's unlikely they will ever gain any sight. Your child is now eighteen months old, and despair sets in as time seems to be running out. Well, that hopelessness ends here. If you begin to stimulate your child's brain in a particular manner, you can significantly develop neuro-connections and encourage a pathway to vision. We know this is possible. We've seen it happen with children who visit our clinic.

What would it take exactly to go from blindness to seeing? Consider the routine of a typical newborn. When that baby wakes up from a long sleep, Mom enters the nursery, turns on the light, and the baby's pupils contract. After Mom changes the baby's diaper and turns off the light, the eyes dilate. Mom then takes the baby downstairs to the brightly lit kitchen and the eyes contract again. Depending on the routine, the baby is exposed to different light reflexes throughout the day until the child is tired. Then it's back to sleep with the lights out again. This scenario probably occurs about fifteen to twenty times a day, and within a few weeks, that baby develops a healthy light reflex. By two and a half weeks, the baby is now starting to see outlines. By two months, the baby can now discern those outlines clearly and consistently. If you calculate it, that "lights on, lights off" stimulation occurs about fifteen times a day—that's just over one hundred times a week, more than four hundred visual stimulations in a month, and more than eight hundred visual pathway stimulations by two months. But if that baby remains in total darkness the whole time, without any light reflex, their neural pathway won't develop, profoundly hindering their vision. Even if they were suddenly placed in a well-lit room, they wouldn't be able to see. They'd be functionally blind.

Babies need stimulation via the contrast between light and dark so that their brains make connections that will help develop healthy vision. Hurt children may need ten times the normal amount of stimulation to promote the development necessary to see in a neurotypical way. While ten times more sounds like a lot, it can be done!

There is a therapy to use for stimulating the visual pathway of a blind child (those with no light reflex). Take this child into a dark room. Then using a bright light—one million candle intensity—stimulate that child's visual pathway for sixty seconds by turning the light on for one second and off for five seconds, for a total cycle of six seconds. Do this ten times in a minute. If you perform this routine twenty to thirty times per day, you'll simulate two to three hundred light on/light off sequences. If you continue this regimen, you could stimulate the visual pathway as many as six to nine thousand times per month. It may seem like a lot—and it is—but the brain requires this type of ongoing stimulation to create the necessary organization to develop. Remember, the brain grows by use, and the function of the stimulation grows the structure of the brain.

Each child is different, as is the origin of each child's challenge. What remains constant is that the process of healing takes intention, attention, and being consistent—in other words, frequency, intensity, and duration. If you're the parent of this blind child, you probably want nothing more than to make this commitment. Maybe you increase your efforts by shining the light forty minutes a day instead of thirty. Or maybe the best you can do is fifteen stimulations per day. If you do whatever you can with consistency, the brain will respond. That's the law of neurodevelopment. This consistent effort will pay off the moment you see the pupils in your child's eyes finally contract and dilate. And achieving that amazing response for the first time will keep you even more hopeful and motivated to continue your efforts: keeping the frequency, intensity, and duration going in order to stimulate the brain, create new pathways, and make further progress.

HOW MUCH STIMULATION IS NEEDED TO PROMOTE DEVELOPMENT?

Regardless of which sensory pathway is compromised—whether vision level one (Seeing and Reading), hearing levels two and three (Hearing and Understanding), tactile levels two and three (Sensation and Tactility), or limbic brain level one (Emotional and Social)—the severity of the injury will determine the amount of stimulation needed. Once you complete the IDPC, you will see exactly where your child is, neurologically, and the degree of their disorganization.

From our clinical experience, we've separated the level of injury into four degrees, each of which needs a different amount of stimulation. These categories correspond with the proficiency assessments noted in the IDPC:

Achieved (A)	No issues
Nearly Achieved (NA)	"Moderate" issue
Partially Achieved (PA)	"Severe" issue
Not Yet Achieved (NYA)	"Profound" issue

Consider the previous example of the child who does not see or even respond to a light reflex. This is considered a profound issue, requiring the highest frequency, intensity, and duration of stimulation. With each greater degree, the stimulation required is more frequent. For example, for a child at seeing and reading level one who is NYA, thirty light stimulations would be ideal. If PA, then twenty light stimulations. If NA, ten should be sufficient.

Overall, we recommend beginning with a frequency that seems to be in line with the degree you have measured your child. If you see positive changes after a month or two, continue until your child is responding well. Then begin to gradually reduce the frequencies. As long as the changes remain, you can wean your child off that stimulation over the course of a month or so. If, however, you're not seeing changes at your initial frequency level, an increase is in order.

STIMULATION FOR DEVELOPING THE SENSORY PATHWAYS

Now that you understand the general principles of frequency, intensity, and duration, and the principle that sensory development will always precede motor competence, we will begin outlining the necessary quantities of sensory stimulation needed to develop a pathway, as a general rule. What follows are sensory activities you can incorporate into your child's daily life that target specific deficits or challenges, and the areas of the brain that control these functions.

When doing these sensory sessions, remember that the more frequency, intensity, and duration you can apply, the more readily you will begin to see your child improve.

Begin with what your child needs the most help with, focusing on only one thing at first. Only add a second focus if you have time and the first stimulation is occurring consistently with the appropriate frequencies. Wait ten to fifteen minutes before repeating the same stimulation session.

If you notice that your child is becoming agitated or emotionally dys-regulated in any session, *stop*. This is your child showing the stimulation was enough and signaling they need a break to integrate the information.

The most common areas in which children need stimulation are detailed in this next section as well. Most of the children we see need one or all of these areas stimulated.

HEARING AND UNDERSTANDING (LEVEL ONE)

Make a series of loud, unexpected sounds by banging a block on a table or banging two blocks together several times. This session can be repeated ten to twenty times daily.

HEARING AND UNDERSTANDING (LEVEL TWO)

Make a sudden, scary, and unexpected sound. Ideas for sounds could be an air horn, stereo, or car horn. To start, we recommend doing this once daily, with a daily *maximum* of three to five times. *Note: Loud sounds must be at a safe distance—across the room, pointed away from the ears of your child and you. Also, you can only do a few of these stimulations in a day or you will damage your and your child's ears over time.*

HEARING AND UNDERSTANDING (LEVEL THREE)

Begin with sounds for the child to learn, locate, and become less sensitive to. You can use many different environmental sounds (bells, whistles, con-tainers you fill, egg shakers, etc.). You can perform ten to twenty sessions per day, with each session lasting one minute. During the session, make three sounds and have your child turn and locate the sounds. You can use the same sounds for a week and then change to something different.

SENSATION AND TACTILITY (LEVEL TWO)

Helping to develop your child's ability to feel pain in their body sufficiently is important for their safety, but you should only do this stimulation if you feel comfortable. You can use toothpicks or ice packs that *won't hurt your child's skin*. Be sure to stimulate only on bare skin. The session should stop as soon as your child begins to respond. If you do not see a response after one minute, stop. Aim for ten to twenty sessions daily. *Note: Be* very *careful not to harm the skin.*

SENSATION AND TACTILITY (LEVEL THREE)

If your child is oversensitive or underreactive to light touches, tickling, or tags in clothes, brushing with textures will be helpful. Choose two contrasting sensations—one semi-rough and one soft—and brush your child's bare skin. Stop if your child becomes agitated. If she is not agitated, you can continue for one minute. Aim for ten to twenty sessions daily. *Note: Be* very *careful not to harm the skin.*

EMOTIONAL AND SOCIAL (LEVEL ONE) (OLFACTORY)

Stimulating the olfactory pathway grows the emotional centers of the brain (limbic system). This can help your child to regulate emotions, become less sensitive to smells in general, and less sensitive to the smells of foods in particular. Stimulating the olfactory pathway can improve eating in picky eaters as the child becomes less sensitive to the smell of the food they eat.

You are looking for your child to react instantly and appropriately to both pleasant and unpleasant smells. You can begin with three smells in a session. Give your child time to take in each smell, and pause between the smells. If the odors are unpleasant, hold them at a distance at first. Over time you will be able to get closer. Repeat the session three times per day. If your child doesn't respond to bad smells, add a stronger smell like nasty fish food. It's *very* important that the smells you use are natural, organic, and chemical-free.

It's good to expose your child to smells that fit the time of day. Generally, morning smells like orange, lime, grapefruit, coffee, peppermint, and lemon should be uplifting, afternoon smells such as rose, lilac, eucalyptus, sage, and cinnamon are comforting, and evening smells like lavender, ylang-ylang, chamomile, and cedarwood are more cozy and downregulating. Using aromatherapy, in addition to the overall stimulation, can be helpful not only for your child but also for you. Some smells can be helpful in specific situations. Rosemary is good for transitioning. Give your child this smell in preparation for a transition or if they get upset over a transition. Smells like rose, rosemary, and lavender can help when a child is upset or out of control with a tantrum.

INTEGRATING STIMULATIONS

Whenever possible, integrate stimulations, so that you cover and involve as many of the senses as possible.

Show your child a picture of a lemon and say, "This is a picture of a lemon." Let your child see and touch a real lemon and say, "This is a lemon." Then let your child smell and taste the lemon.

This type of integrated session exposes your child to one item through all five senses: vision, hearing, touch, taste, and smell.

When your child is awake, stimulate as many senses and functions as possible: visual, auditory, tactile, mobility, and olfactory. After the child sleeps or eats, begin stimulation again with the next function on your list.

SEEING AND READING (LEVEL ONE) (VISION)

The stimulation of the light reflex promotes vision.

If your child's light reflex is zero, incomplete, or inconsistent, then we need to help them develop this pathway. Go into a totally dark room for one minute and turn on a flashlight for one second. Turn it off for five seconds. Repeat ten times. Repeat this session ten, twenty, or thirty times, depending on whether your child is NA, PA, or NYA. *Note: The visual pathway is only stimulated for children who do not yet see and/or have a poor light reflex.*

SEEING AND READING (LEVEL TWO) (VISION)

In these sessions, your child learns to track.

Move a bright-white or colored light (a red bike light works well) *slowly* side to side for your child to follow or find. This is hard work for a child who is learning to see. Therefore, the maximum time per day is ten one- to two-minute sessions. *Note: This session can be done while you are in a dark room stimulating the light reflex session.*

Once a child starts responding to lights, we begin to show them images with black-and-white outlines. Show three different images, one at a time, in a well-lit room. Tell your child what they are seeing as you watch their eyes rest on the picture. Show them the images three to five times per day. Rotate an average of twenty pictures over a few months. You can add more pictures to the day as long as your child is awake enough to see them five times per day.

As with the light, this is hard work for a visually impaired child, so give them a break every three pictures. If your child has seen twenty different black-and-white pictures and is getting bored, you can begin to add some color to the pictures.

Set up the environment with lights and black-and-white on a board or on the wall near them. This gives your child something easy to see and a reason to turn on their vision.

MOVEMENT: THE ESSENTIAL MIND-BODY CONNECTION

We discussed mobility to some extent earlier in the book, but now we're going to go much deeper into the why and how of movement.

Primary medulla reflexes, commando crawling on the belly, creeping on hands and knees, walking, running, and balance activities are essential and the core to the development of the entire brain. Without these normal ontogenetic (the development of a human brain from the medulla through to the cortex) developmental stages occurring robustly, the brain cannot complete its organizational process. In fact, these natural hierarchical ontogenetic movements generate the necessary connections in the brain to allow all seven human functions—Vision and Reading, Hearing and Understanding, Sensation and Tactility, Locomotion and Mobility, Communication and Speech, Manual and Writing, Emotional and Social—to flourish. Again, this principle of ontogenetic neurodevelopment will ultimately foster a child's growth and development into adulthood.

For instance, from a developmental standpoint, if an infant's tonic neck reflex isn't occurring as it should, it's likely the child won't crawl correctly on their belly. And if they don't crawl properly and integrate primary reflexes (and, therefore, properly organize the pons), that ultimately compromises other steps in the developmental process that are necessary for becoming neurologically well organized.

Further, regardless of the state of a child's wellness, there's an unfortunate factor that has affected child development. Over the last forty years, parents have been advised by some physicians, parenting books, the media, and other parents to care for their infants in ways that often curtail movement and, hence, impede neurological development. This occurs, first and foremost, from the moment our babies are born, as we've taken to avoiding placing them on their stomachs. While the idea of putting infants to sleep in a supine position (in other words, on their backs) began decades ago to help prevent sudden infant death syndrome (SIDS), that concept unintentionally led to a drastic decrease in tummy time to the detriment of healthy neurological development.

THE IMPACT OF SIDS

Sudden infant death syndrome (SIDS), also known as crib death, is a baffling and heart-wrenching occurrence resulting in the abrupt and unexplained death of a child under the age of one year, the most critical age being two to four months old. To this day, the exact cause of this condition remains unknown. Speculation has included exposure to tobacco smoke, suffocation, overheating, sleep position, bed sharing, heart issues, low birth weight, and genetic causes.

As a result, in 1994, the American Academy of Pediatrics and the National Institute of Child Health and Human Development began a "Back to Sleep" campaign, advocating that infants should be placed on their backs (supine position) to sleep to reduce the risks of SIDS. Since that time, there has been a significant decrease in the number of SIDS deaths.

In 2011, the campaign was rebranded as "Safe to Sleep" to encompass and educate parents about safe sleep environments. This campaign also recommends and supports the concept of "Tummy Time" for babies during their waking hours to help strengthen head, neck, and shoulder muscles, improve motor skills, and to prevent flattening of the head. (You can learn more at www1.nichd.nih.gov/sts/about/pages/tummytime.aspx.)

The bottom line is to be aware of the risk factors for SIDS, never let a baby sleep prone (on the stomach) on an adult mattress—only a smooth, warm, flat, firm environment—and make time for plenty of supervised tummy time.

THE IMPORTANCE OF THE PRONE POSITION AND ITS IMPACT ON MOVEMENT

When babies are in the uterus, how much are they moving? All the time, right? And if a mother-to-be doesn't feel her baby move for a couple of days, worry sets in, often followed by an immediate visit to the ob-gyn for an examination to ensure everything is okay.

However, once that baby is born, neurological misunderstanding can take over. Suddenly they're immediately placed on their back. This position, sadly, becomes the norm, whether sleeping in a crib or bassinet, or secured in a swing or lounger/floor seat. When removed from a bed or seat, babies are frequently held by Mom or Dad or attached to their bodies via a carrier. Even if they're moved to a blanket on a floor, babies are placed on their backs or beneath an activity gym. There is little opportunity for real body movement, and this results in a neurological disconnect. Some babies are on their backs for so long that their heads get flat and misshapen—some even wind up losing patches of hair on the back of their heads. There are even special helmets now that flat-headed toddlers can wear to reshape the skull, but that doesn't help the brain inside that head.

Even as they grow, most babies are continually placed in play sets, bouncers, jumpers, high chairs, and other stationary contraptions that are colorful, musical, and restricting. Even though these all may provide peace of mind—that our children are safe and content—our babies are missing the opportunity to *move*, to turn on their brains, and make vital neural connections that encourage proper neurodevelopment and wellness.

If you put your baby on his stomach on a clean, smooth, hard surface either near your bed or on a firm protective mat on the floor of your living room, that baby will have the opportunity to crawl three or four feet on the first day of his life. Why? Because babies are hardwired to move. Further, when a baby is in the prone position, they breathe deeper, sleep more deeply (healthy for the brain), and they also release potential gas and congestion.

Imagine you are on a flight from New York to Tokyo and you can't move around, even if you are served excellent meals and drinks, watch an endless array of movies, and catch a nap. Fourteen-plus hours later, when you get off the plane, you will be achy or numb and probably a little constipated. It's no different for our babies. They go from the bed to a seat or stroller. They are carried around and then put on their backs again so that there's no chance to move. And what happens? They get cranky, fussy, and even colicky. For babies, toddlers, kids, teenagers, and adults, the more we move, the better we function physiologically and neurologically.

You have probably witnessed babies crying when they are placed on their tummies—it seems like an automatic function. Stomach = crying. But babies *want* to move. Moving is how we all initially survive and later thrive.

If you put the baby on a mat on the floor, they will eventually cry. But if you give them a little time, you'll see them start to move. Most of the time this cry isn't one of sadness or sleepiness (because most babies cry for these reasons *before* you put them down), but a cry akin to the grunt of an athlete running or a teenager putting considerable effort into a sport. If you encourage many short distances of movement, placing your hands behind their feet so they can use them to propel forward, the infant will learn. The more they move, the more they learn, and the more the brain develops.

If, however, we get confused or concerned about our child's crying and immediately pick them up to comfort them, we can unintentionally reinforce the opposite—that movement is difficult, and that Mom and Dad are responsible for their movement. We want you to encourage mobility independence, not dependence.

It's not just the neurology that benefits from movement, it's overall physical and physiological health. A baby that moves is developing the structure of their joints and the balance of flexors and extensors—their muscles! Therefore, the principle that *function determines structure* is in full view. A baby in correct ontogenetic motion grows into a toddler that develops keen brain function.

We want all children to be moving whether they are hurt or not because when they move well, they gain appropriate respiratory development, nerve conduction, blood and lymphatic circulation, digestion, and elimination. They also develop a healthy physical structure—good hips, spine, neck, ankles—and they move well and effortlessly. Movement fires up and integrates the reflexes, which, in turn, help develop an organized medulla and pons. The pons, as you may recall, is responsible for commando crawling and a multitude of other vital neurological functions including lateral eye movements, tongue control, autonomic regulation, breathing, and sleeping deeply.

Give children ample, organized, and reinforced tummy time every day. Observe them as they explore their world, use their arms, their toes, their limbs, and begin to crawl. Let them move!

CRAWLING AND CREEPING: BACK TO THE FUTURE

Back to the Future is one of our favorite movies of all time, and its title fits well here. We can't say enough about the necessity and benefits of commando crawling. The reason we say "back to the future" is that going back to this most basic of movements is an essential pathway toward promoting increased neurodevelopment for our children, whatever their medical or developmental needs.

Crawling on the belly stimulates the reticular formation/reticular activating system and integrates medullary reflexes that allow children to hold their urine so they don't wet their bed when they're ten. Crawling supports the bowels and bowel movement, and enhances digestion, focus, filtering, tongue movement, side-to-side eye tracking, and facial and cranial nerves—which, in turn, support health and neurological growth. Crawling on the belly governs more than twenty vital functions.

To put it simply, consider this quote from one of our mentors: "The floor is the most expensive piece of equipment you need to heal your child's brain." If you place your child stomach down on the floor and get them to crawl for one hundred days, you're going to start to see a change for the better. Kids that never commando crawled—and there are many of them—will not be able to function adequately because they are not able to organize their neurological hard drive. You complete the organization of a child's hard drive—the brain stem, primarily—through the mobility pathway.

The pons is designed to house specific neurological abilities that cannot adequately develop unless you crawl. And it's part of the natural physical process. Babies left in the prone position on a flat surface would crawl on their bellies (like in the crib at night). Then they would eventually get up and creep on their hands and knees. Finally, they would stand up and walk—all with structural and neurological integrity.

As we have mentioned in earlier chapters, crawling on the belly also helps develop the facial nerves. Ever see a two-month-old child smiling in their sleep? They're not dreaming about their next meal. Those facial movements will eventually help them communicate using expressions. The face expresses more emotion than speech or words. When people converse with you, you believe their face, not their words or tone.

You now have the remarkable opportunity to go back, reorganize, and paint a new neurological future for your child. Regardless of age, if your child starts to crawl, their organized function will appear and increase. Their tracking, filtering, focus, structure, tongue and face movement, and many other functions will all begin to improve. Their hips will move better, as will their shoulders. Coordination, strength, and functions such as bladder and bowel control will improve. There are kids whose arms and legs are splayed or crossed because they didn't move properly enough to develop their reflexes and create an organized skeletal structure where their feet, ankles, hips, spine, shoulders, and neck work together as an integrated team. These kids can be helped, too.

CRAWLING INTO CREEPING

In the evolution of child development, babies naturally go from crawling to creeping. What's the difference? Crawling occurs when infants have enough practice and organization and overcome gravity to pull themselves forward. Creeping begins once babies can defy gravity, lift their stomachs off the floor, support their body over their arms, and move around on their hands and knees. In each case, they are meeting a new level of development of their bodies and their brains.

When a child can crawl correctly, they will easily and naturally progress to the creeping position and begin to creep on their hands and knees. As we pointed out previously, some infants skim over this developmental stage, creep awkwardly late, and pay the consequences later.

We live in a time where the emphasis seems to be to get a child to walk. Our role here is to follow the IDPC chart and to allow your child the maximum amount of time to master their ability to crawl and then to creep. Once they can crawl with consistent toe digging (Babinski reflex in a cross pattern) and creep in a cross pattern well, they are naturally going to stand in the middle of the floor and walk with confidence. To the best of our ability, the objective is to respect the natural path of human neurology and the encouragement of brain growth. If you try to walk your child when they're not yet organized correctly in the brain stem, there is less possibility that they are going to become a proficient and confident walking and running superhero.

If a hurt child has not been able to develop this part of the brain on their own, or while in various therapies has not been given the opportunity to develop these parts of the brain, it will be a challenge for them to make the leap to appropriate walking. They're not going to have the hips for it. They're not going to have the reflexes for it. They're not going to have the organization for it. They're going to need to use a walker, and that's not walking.

If your child is not successfully crawling, you must put a comprehensive plan in place to make this possible. Integrated reflexes plus opportunity begets crawling; ample opportunity to crawl begets creeping on hands and knees; ample creeping on hands and knees begets solid walking; lots of walking begets running.

If an infant or immobile child spends 80 percent of the time crawling, you're focusing on what they can do; that leaves 20 percent of the time for encouraging them to get on all fours to prepare to reach the next level of neurology, which is creeping. When they hit that milestone, they can spend 80 percent of the time creeping on their hands and knees, standing, and walking in a cross pattern. Then, when they start to walk, 80 percent of the time will be dedicated to walking and then 20 percent toward helping them run. This is the way you build (or rebuild) their neurology and reflexes. You encourage your child's progress from crawling on their belly to creeping on their hands and knees, to walking and to running, and then, anything else they may want to do physically, whether ice skating, skiing, ballroom dancing, wrestling, football, or basketball. We invent ways to enjoy our mobility all the time—it is part of our human experience.

The more crawling and creeping, the more the brain will grow. Physically, crawling provides structure and fosters strong hips, ankles, feet, and shoulders. Creeping improves coordination and the ability to replicate functions, move in a graceful cross pattern, and develop convergence and depth perception.

If you survey the parents of a class of first graders who have trouble with focus and attention, you will probably discover that most of those children probably never crawled or crept. So it is imperative that, regardless of age, current limitations, or labels, you must begin to get your child moving in the most ontogenetic developmental manner as soon as you possibly can.

Going forward, remember that mobility is the most complex function of the brain.

- The function of reflexes develops and organizes the medulla.
- The function of crawling develops and organizes the pons.
- The function of creeping develops and organizes the midbrain.
- The function of vestibular activities develops and matures the cerebellum.
- The function of walking and running develops and organizes the cortex.

Returning to the lower levels of the brain via reflexes, crawling, and creeping promotes substantial brain growth for disorganized children who are walking.

THE BASIC BRAIN ORGANIZATION PROGRAM

If your child is mobile but struggling with attention, focus, language, visual tracking, convergence, depth perception, organization, coordination, regulation, or hyper- or hyposensitivity, the following program is important for helping your child gain those important functions.

GUIDELINES FOR SUCCESS

- Clothing
  - Your child should wear comfortable, loose-fitting clothes in which they can move around with ease.

- Safety
  - Protect your child's knees and elbows with padding and good quality mats, if necessary.

- Environment
  - Children should start this program on a smooth surface and graduate to a carpeted surface. It is unwise to do this outside directly on the grass.
  - Ensure that the environment in which you work with your child is:
    » clean
    » safe
    » consistent
    » spacious/long
    » fun

- Motivation
  - Children who can crawl and creep, and who are doing this as part of a program to improve neurological organization, need to be motivated differently than children who need to move as a way of life.
  - Create a fun, personal, homemade book with relevant pictures your child can relate to and write in all the specific objectives, environment, dynamics, goals, and rewards. This makes it very clear to the child what he can expect from you, and what you expect from him.
  - Acknowledge children for their efforts with immediate rewards such as hugs, books, and toys.

- Rewards
  - You can award your child with tokens when completing each session.
  - As the day progresses, he can redeem these tokens for rewards such as playing, watching a video, learning, reading, and playing with friends.
  - Your child needs the opportunity to earn frequent daily, weekly, and some monthly rewards.
  - Gaining these rewards teaches your child that cooperation and success leads to free time and many privileges.
  - As they make noticeable strides in intellectual development, reward your child with tokens, points, or money for completing the task. Give bonuses for attitude, speed, and independence.
  - Children also learn the value of saving and delaying gratification.

- How to Succeed
  - Structure your program. Using the fun, upbeat, organized homemade book, make it clear to your child what you expect and what he can expect, too. Stick to the structure as best you can. The more disorganized your child, the more structure he will need to succeed. In our experience, the more a child can anticipate the next step, the happier he will be.
  - Do it together. Engage together. As much as possible, have family members participate in these activities alongside your child.
  - Conduct these activities in a clean, open, and well-lit area. Have gym mats well positioned and construct the track throughout the home for as long as it can go. The longer the track, the more interesting it will be for your child.
  - Five-finger toe shoes are great as they enable the child to use his entire foot to crawl by pushing off his feet, using the big toe as an anchor. Kneepads and elbow pads are a must if your

child is heavier than sixty pounds. You may want to attach
these pads into the clothing for more flexibility.

– Spread out the physical activities in between the sensory and
learning opportunities.

– Start slowly and progressively build up to the distances you
want your child to achieve over time.

– Organize rewards according to the combined average of
your child's intellectual and social age. For instance, if your
child is ten years old chronologically but four years old
neurologically, immediate detailed feedback and rewards
are necessary. If your child is twelve years old with a neurological age of eight, money may motivate him to meet his
distance goals.

SAMPLE PROGRAM

What follows are the basic movement exercises we recommend you
implement so that you can begin making strides in your child's brain
organization.

- *Crawling*
  - Ideal length: Two hundred meters (650 feet) of crawling.
  - Amount: Begin by crawling ten times per day, four meters
    (thirteen feet) per session. Each week, increase the crawling
    by two meters (6.5 feet) per week until your child is crawling
    ten times per day, twenty meters (sixty-five feet) nonstop
    per session, for a total of two hundred meters (650 feet) per
    day. Over the next six weeks, reduce to four times a day but
    increase each session to fifty meters (164 feet).
  - Environment: Smooth. Use mats or carpet.

- *Creeping*
  - Ideal length: One kilometer (3,280 feet) of creeping.

- Amount: Begin by creeping ten times per day, ten meters (thirty-two feet) per session, one hundred meters (328 feet) nonstop per session, for a total of one thousand meters (one kilometer or 3,280 feet) per day. Gradually increase this to five sessions a day at two hundred meters (650 feet) each.
- Environment: Smooth. Use mats or carpet.

ADDITIONAL GUIDELINES

- Create a fun obstacle course of tunnels, elevated mats, and cones to crawl and creep through and around.
- Spread the sessions out over the course of each day.
- Most importantly, enjoy the time with your child and make it fun.

FACTORS TO CONSIDER WHEN CREATING A PLAN FOR YOUR CHILD

When creating a plan for your child, there are several important factors to consider:

- Evaluate and measure. We've impressed upon you the need to assess and understand exactly where your child is today, developmentally. You can't have a plan if you don't know your child's status and the developmental milestones you hope they will eventually reach. Once you measure your child's abilities, your plan should encompass the steps necessary to take them where they need to go. You will need to integrate therapies, exercises, and tools that specifically target the areas of your child's brain that need attention.
- You now understand your child better and know more of what they need and what it will take to achieve that. With that knowledge and the necessary tools and time, you'll be able to create a plan and proactively stick to it. That will, in turn, give you a sense of how to create a schedule that balances the time you have to

work with your child with all the other things you have to do daily: tend to the rest of your family, run errands, keep appointments, and have "me" time.

- You should try to strike a balance between the sensory, motor areas, and social skills for a well-rounded approach. You accomplish this by referring to the IDPC chart. The chart will guide your focus on the areas you need to address and ensure that you don't overlook some things or spend too much time on areas you shouldn't. A good balance would be to spend 80 percent of your time on the things that are the most vital, 10 to 15 percent of the time on things that are important, and 5 percent of the time on things that are helpful but not critical. However, anything less than 80 percent spent toward critical areas may increase the time it takes to reach a goal. There are many ways to create a formula that combines what is necessary with what is practical and recreational. Be creative. Keep everything in balance.
- Understand the difference between physiology and pathology.
- Be consistent.
- Be very patient with your child and yourself. It takes time to shift and integrate this neurodevelopmental approach into your child's—and your—daily life.
- Be organized. Organization supports execution. Execution with joy brings prosperity and drives development.
- Assess results regularly. Gauge the results. Every three months, look at the goals you reached (or didn't quite meet) and revise the plan accordingly.

DESIGNING YOUR CHILD'S NEURODEVELOPMENT PLAN

When creating your child's program, keep the following in mind:

- Use the IDPC chart to decide what is needed to change your child.

- Decide on the frequency, intensity, and duration of sensory and motor stimulation your child needs for change to occur.
- Prioritize what skills you work on first, second, third, etc.
- Make a checklist or create a notebook in which material can be rearranged.
- Start with one thing at a time.
- Use a timer to remind you when it is time for your next allocated session.
- Add a little more to your sessions each day.
- Once you are consistent with one element, begin adding the next aspect of the program.

FAMILY SUCCESS STORY

Greetings from South Africa! I attended the PTC in February this year. With her first evaluation I did at the parent training conference, our daughter was neurologically two and a half years behind her chronological age, and she was at 70 percent degree of function. For six months we only did the FHC program and reflex integration of five reflexes that were still active. We also had three craniosacral sessions. I evaluated her again after three months on the program and was astonished at the improvement she'd shown. (Not to mention the difference we'd already seen in her behavior, emotions, and actions at that point!)

I did her six-month reevaluation recently, and at first, I didn't expect there'd be much more improvement, but when I'd finished, I was in awe! Her neurological age has caught up with her chronological nine years of age completely, and she is at 99 percent degree of function!

Last year we were told that her challenges were due to her "wiring" and that we could do nothing about it. We were told, "She 'needs to learn to cope with it.'"

Today, a year later, all those challenges are a thing of the past. She again is the happy, flourishing girl we had lost during the last few years. And our family has completely healed.

None of this would have been possible if it wasn't for Matthew and Carol. I would not have known about you if it wasn't for one other mom and the Brain Child Fund's information session last year. I am eternally grateful to our Lord for bringing us to you, so that our daughter could be healed.

Because of this, I have been spreading this good news as far and wide as possible, so that more children and their families can heal. Thank you for doing what you do with so much drive and enthusiasm! Thank you so much for empowering us as parents to be the necessary "assistive devices" to our children in their lives.

—*Ananda and Banie van der Walt*

NEURO-PARENTING POINTS

- The brain grows physically with stimulation—this is the principle of neuroplasticity, which is the ability of the brain to adapt and change. This occurs in response to stimulation, by making new connections, and by laying down new pathways.
- The process of developing and honing neurological abilities takes frequency, intensity, and duration, which is achieved by movement—the essential mind/body connection.
- The most basic and natural movement is crawling. Babies that crawl on their stomachs exhibit greater neurotypical development—and overall improved physical and physiological health—than those that do not. Remember, function determines structure—the brain's neural network matures as well as the structure of the body—more organized joints and stronger muscles.

- The floor is the most expensive piece of equipment you need to heal your child's brain. Regardless of age or abilities, encouraging your child to crawl will help to improve brain function because the brain grows by use.
- Crawling on the belly (commando crawling) leads to creeping on hands and knees. Creeping, in turn, leads to walking and then running. The more crawling and creeping, the more the brain will grow. These basic levels of mobility will improve and strengthen physical movement and organization.
- Create an environment that is conducive to fostering movement. Dress your child comfortably, protect their knees and elbows, and provide a clean, smooth, and safe environment in which they can move.
- Work with your child daily and consistently. As they improve, add more time and distance to movement and activities to meet new levels of proficiency.
- Reward your child along the way to reinforce and motivate their efforts.

CHAPTER 7

CARE AND NOURISHMENT OF YOUR CHILD

Here's some food for thought: as professionals in the field of child development, we really cannot stress enough the value and impact that a wholesome diet of water and food—along with a healthy environment—can have on the development of your child and your family.

Children with special needs struggle physiologically. They have unique sensitivities to food, their environment, and anything related to the five senses—touch, taste, vision, hearing, and smell—all of which are seemingly acute. Watching your child, we're sure you're already aware how even minor environmental changes affect your and their emotions, mood, attention span, sleep, digestion, and overall health. We encourage you to pay serious and consistent attention to how your child is nourished. Their brain desperately needs quality nutrition to develop and thrive.

Optimum health, simply put, is achieved by the body's ability to collect and distribute energy successfully. The sources through which we gather that energy include air, water, food, exercise, sleep, environment, and contact with people. All of these sources of energy can be either nutritious or toxic, depending on how or where they are obtained and their quality level.

AIR

Clean air and oxygen are of vital importance for your child's success. In fact, 21 percent of the air we breathe is oxygen, and oxygen is the primary food for the brain. Most of the time, brain injury occurs when the brain suffers a significant loss of oxygen. Anoxia (the absence of oxygen) causes the injury; hypoxia (insufficient oxygen) compounds the damage.

In addition to oxygen, carbon dioxide is necessary because it regulates the blood flow. Carbon dioxide helps absorb oxygen properly, and there should be a balance between oxygen and carbon dioxide in a child's system. The brain uses about 30 to 50 percent of all oxygen and nutrients from the blood, so enhancing blood flow to the brain increases the delivery of vital nutrition. Physical activity improves blood flow.

When the weather and circumstances are favorable, take your child outdoors for some fresh air. Going outdoors improves heart rate and blood pressure, helps eliminate any impurities from the lungs, boosts the immune system, sharpens the mind, and increases energy. Further, exposure to natural sunlight helps provide vitamin D, which is essential.

When you can't get outside, ensure that there is clean air inside the house—air that's free from mold and mildew. Mold and mildew are harmful to the brain's ability to function. To improve air quality, open the windows and air out the house. Clean up dust, pet hair, and other dirt with natural products and vacuums with HEPA filters. Be sure to clean out air conditioner filters and air ducts on a regular basis. Avoid the use of air fresheners and cleaning products other than those made from natural ingredients (there are many easy-to-find online resources for making natural cleaning products at home inexpensively). Investing in an indoor air purifier is also worthwhile because it helps to eliminate many types of germs and pollutants.

WATER

The consumption of pure water is the number-one nutritional objective for your child's journey to wellness. Water maintains all vital body functions, including synthesis of adenosine triphosphate (ATP) to run the cells and provide hydration, lymph drainage, cerebral fluid, and the nourishment of fascia. In fact, water is vital to the health and optimal function of the brain as well as the peripheral nervous system, including the production of hormones and neurotransmitters.

That's not surprising, really, considering that water is a primary constituent of every cell in the body. Even the space between cells is composed primarily of water. A newborn's body is 75 percent water; by age one, it's 65 percent water. And the brain itself is 75 to 85 percent water. Consistent hydration supplies nutrients to the brain, which increase cognitive function, concentration, clarity, and memory.

If your child's body and brain are insufficiently hydrated or even dehydrated, it can trigger a chain reaction of symptoms related to mental and physical fatigue resulting in brain fog, erratic emotions, sleep problems, and an array of digestive issues. In fact, in our clinical experience, many children who are neurologically compromised frequently lack proper hydration, which further compounds the injury in the brain.

Proper biochemistry, detoxification, and elimination require an abundant supply of filtered water. To ensure access to pure water, consider adding a filtration system to the kitchen faucet, at the very least. Chlorine and fluoride, which are prevalent in the water supply of most US cities (unless you use well water), affect the natural microbial content of the intestines and the nervous and endocrine systems of the body. At a minimum, these chemicals need to be removed.

While breast milk (from a well-nourished mother) is the ideal food/beverage for infants, pure water is the ideal beverage for children—and parents, too. To determine how much water your child requires, take your child's weight (as expressed in pounds of body weight) and divide it in half to get the number of ounces of water per day recommended for the average individual to support basic life functions. For example, a thirty-pound child needs at least fifteen ounces (about a half quart or liter) of water a day. If he or she sweats a lot, is detoxing, or constipated, more water is needed (for metric use: one kilogram = 2.2 pounds and one ounce = 30 ml).

FOOD

The brain consumes more than 20 percent of the body's daily nutrition. Therefore, proper nutrition is critical to superb brain function. How and what we eat—and how our children eat—greatly influences health throughout childhood, adolescence, and adulthood. There is never a moment that your brain and body do not need the absolute best nutrition to optimally function. Of course, none of us eats perfectly all the time, but if we are *mindful* of this concept—particularly for our children who are struggling—we do them a great service.

Food provides the proteins, fats, enzymes, minerals, vitamins, and sugars necessary for proper development. If you understand the value of this concept and are consistent and conscientious about feeding, your child will make significant strides in neurodevelopment. We have seen these results firsthand.

Fats and essential fatty acids are necessary to support the myelin sheath responsible for proper transmission of neural impulses and maintenance of cell membranes. Proteins are necessary to support the neurons, dendrites, muscles, hormones, blood, antibodies, organs, and enzymes—in fact, all cells in the body need proteins. Even carbohydrates and sugars provide energy and some structure.

Given their sensitivities, many children with special needs require a tailored nutritional regimen. You may have noticed this with your child. Others may only need to follow what we consider to be a healthy, nourishing program that would benefit all children in the family (as well as the adults). What follows are basic guidelines that we consider to be important for all families.

This type of mindful nourishment is considered "natural food" or "whole food nutrition." You may already be eating in this manner. If not, it may mean making substantial dietary changes.

Today's modern diet emphasizes speed, convenience of sourcing and preparation, and taste. This often results in meals with high amounts of sugar, refined carbohydrates, refined salt, and unhealthy oils at the expense of real nutrition. Obviously, with multiple family members at home, shifting to a natural, organic, low-glycemic, water-based hydration focus might not be easy to accomplish. But the truth is that this is a valuable action to take. It will help your child progress if you can be consistent, so find the support system to begin making such changes.

If you fall into the "speed and convenience" group, try to make changes step by step. Start by eliminating the worst of the foods and beverages that your family consumes on a regular basis and replace them with options that are truly nourishing and helpful to the body.

You may need to treat this change as a new skill to be learned. We also strongly recommend creating a weekly menu so you can plan your meals and grocery shopping in advance. Having the whole family—and extended family members—committed to this nutrition program will also be helpful or even vital to its success.

Keep in mind that it's easier for *everyone* in your family to adopt a new eating plan than to alter the diet of your child with special needs alone. And everyone will reap the benefits from healthy eating and improved nutrition.

EATING TOGETHER

All children and families benefit from the fellowship of eating together in a peaceful, TV-free, cell phone–free environment. When done regularly, or at least whenever possible, this daily activity builds stronger family relationships and healthier eating habits for everyone. If your child can learn to sit comfortably at the table and among the family, consider the ideal goal met.

However, if you find that you need to put 100 percent of your attention toward your child's eating due to feeding and behavioral reasons, such a mealtime dynamic may not be practical. Our advice is to feed your child first—and to do so mindfully—and then bring them to the table for a few minutes (or for as long as they are comfortable) to be part of the family meal. As they acclimate, you can increase that time spent at the table and even begin integrating some food.

Another helpful strategy is to get your child involved and engaged in preparing the meal. There are many ways to accomplish this, from taking them grocery shopping to having them help prep some of the food. If you have a vegetable, fruit, or herb garden, take your child into the yard and let them be involved, even if they just watch you care for the plants or gather up veggies for that night's meal. Setting the table together, tasting the food together, or just having your child watch you buzz around the kitchen cooking will all help your child see the value of food and nutrition, enhance their sense of smell, and foster the connection around meals in your family.

BASIC NUTRITION GUIDELINES

When figuring out how to make changes to best support your child's development and health, it can be useful to have a few basic guidelines to work from. Here's our take.

Decrease the Consumption of Processed and Refined Foods

The first objective of good nutrition is to markedly decrease the amount of processed and refined foods and increase the amount of food prepared at home and composed of ingredients that are organic and/or natural, whole, fresh, and as free of chemicals as possible.

The quality of the food is of primary importance. Eating nourishes the cells of the body and provides them with the high-quality energy to perform their many functions. These include the cells of the brain, nervous system, vital organs, muscles, and bones. Each of these specialized tissues has a specific job to do and requires certain nutrients to do that job. Eating a wide variety of fresh, natural, unadulterated, and minimally processed foods is the best way to obtain more than one hundred different nutrients that our body requires regularly to achieve that optimal functionality.

Imagine the kinds of food that were available to a non-impoverished family living about one hundred years ago. Fresh, seasonal vegetables and fruits were grown locally without the use of pesticides and artificial fertilizers. Eggs, poultry, fish, and meat came from animals raised in their natural environments, eating their natural food, without the use of growth-stimulating hormones and antibiotics. Loaves of bread and cereals were made from whole grains, without artificial flavorings, colors, and man-made fats (like hydrogenated oils). And, of course, pure water.

This type of diet contains minimally processed foods. The processing or refining of food—which generally takes place in a facility between the farm where it is grown or raised and the home where it is consumed—almost always results in the depletion of essential nutrients like fiber, minerals, and vitamins. These are replaced with artificial substances (like hydrogenated oils, synthetic dyes, artificial flavors, preservatives, and sweeteners) that interfere with the body's normal functioning. Examples of processed and refined foods include white flour, white rice, canned vegetables and fruits, dried and powdered foods (like macaroni and cheese in a box or artificial creamer), snack foods (like candy bars, potato chips, cookies, etc.), and most food items that come in packages with a label full of ingredients.

Natural foods—foods that are as close as possible to the way they are found in nature, and with no labels—will have the highest nutrient content and an absence of artificial substances. These are referred to as "whole foods." A whole grain like whole wheat or brown rice will contain substantially more fiber, minerals, and vitamins than refined grains like white wheat flour or white rice. The general caution is to avoid "white foods" as these highly processed and refined foods have a low nutrient content, and, usually—because of the lack of fiber—a high glycemic index, which results in unstable blood sugar and insulin levels.

Chemical-free foods are more likely to be found among natural, whole foods due to the absence of artificial additives that are often included in the preparation and packaging of highly processed and refined products. Many commercial growers use various amounts and types of chemicals.

Organic foods—those that are grown or raised the old-fashioned way without the use of pesticides and artificial fertilizers—are a healthier choice. For a long time, you could only purchase organic foods at health food or specialty stores, but now they are regularly available at most national supermarket chains. Most supermarkets even have aisles devoted exclusively to organic and wholesome foods. When buying organic, most products are labeled with a green "USDA Organic" seal, though smaller producers don't require this label (in which case, double-check the status with the produce manager). The options can include local food co-ops, farmers' markets, and shopping online for home delivery.

Of equal, if not greater, importance than buying organic produce is seeking out and purchasing hormone-free and antibiotic-free animal-based foods such as beef, chicken, eggs, and dairy products. The factory farms in which most of these food sources are raised—particularly in the US—routinely use steroidal, growth-enhancing hormones to increase muscle mass and egg and milk volume.

Antibiotics are included in the feed to prevent common infections that often materialize in the crowded and unnatural living conditions of the animals. These chemicals can be absorbed by the animals that are the source of the meat we eat, which means we ingest these chemicals, too.

Farm-raised fish and seafood pose another set of problems due to other chemicals that make their way into the bodies of those fish. There are no safe and healthy fish-farming practices, so you must be informed about this source of food as well. In general, it is preferable to select wild fish over farm-raised fish. Small-sized wild fish are recommended.

Mercury is a toxic metal that has found its way into most bodies of water in the world due to pollution. Purchasing mercury-free fish is another important consideration. Your children may already have problems with a buildup of toxic metals in their bodies, so avoid adding to that burden. Generally, the smaller the size of the fish, the less likely the presence of mercury in its tissues. According to EWG.org (more details in the sidebar on the following page), the fish and shellfish that are highest in omega-3 and lowest in mercury are:

- Salmon (wild)
- Sardines
- Mussels
- Rainbow trout
- Atlantic mackerel
- Oysters
- Pollock
- Herring

Other toxic metals and substances can be found in various foods. Arsenic, for example, is routinely added to the feed of most chickens raised in factory farms, but that does not apply to chickens raised organically. Though buying organically raised food is not an absolute guarantee that it's free of chemicals (chemicals can enter the plant or animal via contaminated or polluted water), overall, the incidence of toxic substances is considerably less and the nutrient content significantly higher when you purchase organically raised foods.

Unadulterated means that the food was not irradiated or genetically altered (GMO)—two additional ways in which our natural food is transformed or manipulated from its original form. Many researchers and scientists do not believe that these new, man-made molecules are compatible with normal human biochemistry.

Fresh produce has the highest nutrient content and taste appeal. The shorter the time between harvest and consumption, the higher the nutrient content. Fresh-picked, locally grown vegetables and fruits are the most desirable. If there is a local farmers' market in your area, this would be an excellent place to purchase fresh produce. Select a "rainbow" of foods. The more vibrant the color of the fruit or vegetable (such as dark, leafy greens like kale or collards, and blueberries), the higher the overall nutrient content.

If you cannot always buy fresh organic, then frozen produce is an acceptable option. Today's methods use quick-freezing of recently picked fruits and vegetables that result in the retention of high nutrient content. Conversely, canned fruits and vegetables have a low nutrient content, so we suggest that you avoid these. Dried or dehydrated fruits and vegetables should be used in moderation because they can be quite high in sugar and starches. Ideally, it is preferable to eat a piece of fresh fruit rather than a handful of dried fruit.

PESTICIDE RESIDUE IN FOOD

Pesticides, which are known to contribute to a variety of health-related issues, are a significant issue to be mindful of if consuming conventionally grown produce. Research conducted by the Environmental Working Group's analysis of tests by the US Department of Agriculture showed that almost 70 percent of produce samples tested were contaminated with pesticide residue.

What does this mean for the health of you and your child? Ongoing consumption of high-residue produce can cause long-term damage, even in subtle ways, so be aware of what you buy and feed your child.

Will washing and peeling help? Yes and no. Rinsing reduces but does not eliminate pesticides. Peeling helps, but valuable nutrients within the skin will be lost. The best option is to buy organic whenever possible and to rinse all produce well regardless of how it is grown.

Environmental Working Group (EWG) is a nonprofit organization dedicated to protecting human health as well as the environment.

EWG research shows that people who eat five fruits and vegetables a day from their "Dirty 12" list of produce containing high-pesticide residue consume an average of ten pesticides a day. Those who eat from the "Clean 15" list of the fifteen least contaminated, conventionally grown fruits and vegetables ingest fewer than two pesticides daily.

How do you know which fruits and vegetables make each list? Every year, EWG releases their *Shopper's Guide to Pesticides in Produce,* which helps consumers make informed choices to lower their dietary pesticide load. You can review or download these lists by visiting the EWG website at www.ewg.org/foodnews.

The Importance of Regular Mealtimes

The second guideline: ensure your child eats *three* proper meals a day, with one or two healthy snacks between meals. Depending upon the age and needs of your child, it may be necessary to increase to four to five small meals a day.

As you may already know, breakfast is the most important meal of the day. Breakfast—with ample healthy fats and some proteins, to put the brain in a ketogenic state (whereby the body burns fats rather than burning carbs)—provides the energy and the focus needed to have a productive day. Lunch is the second most important meal. Again, protein, along with some good fat and fiber from desirable carbohydrates, will provide lasting energy during those hours of the day when it is most needed. An easy way to determine the quantity of necessary protein per meal is an amount approximately equal to the size of your child's palm. A balanced meal (with adequate protein, fat, and fiber) should provide your child with three to five hours of energy and the absence of hunger. You can plan the timing of meals and snacks in advance and incorporate them into your child's day.

As far as vegetables are concerned, provide as many as possible. Twice as many vegetables as protein is a good rule of thumb. Aim for serving as many colors of vegetables as you can every day.

If your child does not have difficulty digesting food, include a starchy carbohydrate with the meal. Choose cooked whole grains like quinoa, millet, amaranth, and buckwheat as healthy alternatives to rice and wheat; sweet potatoes or yams; and winter squash such as butternut, acorn, and pumpkin. However, these starchy carbohydrates should not be the largest category of food served at the meal, but rather prepared as a side dish.

Fresh, organic raw fruit makes an ideal snack if given in moderation. Some children will eat a lot of fruit, and this can drive their brain to a sugar high and lead to irritable and disorganized behavior. This is one major reason we suggest wholeheartedly that you avoid giving children fruit juice. It contains highly concentrated fructose sugar. If your child can eat

MICROWAVE OVENS

There's no doubt that the microwave oven is a convenient and time-saving invention that is a fixture in most kitchens. However, at this time, there have been many contrasting studies about the effects of microwaves used in food preparation. Some studies suggest that it is fine to microwave food while others strongly recommend avoiding the use of microwaves altogether. Our opinion is: *Why take any risk when it comes to your child?* We believe that water and foods heated with microwaves are depleted in vitality and nutrition. As water naturally warms by both the sun and by fire, we recommend using the stovetop or a toaster oven to cook or warm up food. Though a minimal amount of additional time will be needed to prepare or reheat your food, we adhere to the law of "do no harm." For more information, visit www.emwatch.com/microwave-oven-radiation/.

dairy, a natural, whole-fat, plain yogurt combines very well with the fruit. You can make a smoothie from the yogurt and fruit as an alternative to eating it out of a dish. Nuts and seeds, or natural nut butter made from them, also combine well with fruit. The protein and good fat in the nuts/ seeds and the yogurt will make the snack more of a mini-meal and tide the child over to the next meal better than fruit alone. Again, try to offer a variety of fruits, vegetables, nuts, and seeds.

Consumption of Liquids

As mentioned earlier in this chapter, water should be the primary beverage served to your child. You can occasionally supplement with other drinks.

While less likely to contain artificial ingredients, 100 percent organic fruit juice still has a lot of sugar. Even when labeled as "natural," one glass of orange or apple juice may contain as much sugar as an equal amount of soda. That's a lot of sugar to enter the body at one time.

If your child is accustomed to drinking juice, it is healthier to dilute it with pure water in a ratio of three-parts juice to one-part water. After two or three weeks of serving this to your child, you move to a 2:1 dilution, and then continue until the mixture is one-part juice to three-parts water. If you have a juicer, freshly squeezed vegetable juice can be nutritious, but keep the sweet vegetables like beets and carrots to half or less of the total amount. Eventually, it would be ideal to drink water and have fruit as a snack, prepared in the manner described above.

Some fruit juices have exceptional antioxidant and other properties that can be worthwhile. Among them are blueberry, cranberry, black currant, noni, pomegranate, and mango juices. These should be purchased without added sugar, and again, diluted to avoid fluctuations in blood-sugar levels.

For children with brain injuries, herbal teas with just a bit of natural sweetener are acceptable, as they are high in antioxidants.

Curtailing Sugar Intake

Reducing and eventually eliminating sugar intake is another factor to consider in supporting the health of your child's brain. By avoiding processed and refined foods and beverages, you will already have significantly decreased the amount of sugar entering your child's body. If you don't have a habit of eating desserts or sweetened foods and beverages on a regular basis at home, there shouldn't be a problem with sugar intake for the average child (although some children are sensitive to even small amounts of sugars).

Stevia, a natural sweetener, is extracted from the leaves of the stevia plant. It tastes sweet and is a worthy substitute for sugar. You can purchase it at health food stores in liquid (generally the most useful) or in powder form. Stevia can be used safely by almost everyone, including those with blood-sugar control problems and overgrowth of undesirable organisms, such as yeast, in the intestines.

Honey (especially raw, unfiltered, and not subjected to high heat) and date sugar are examples of natural choices of sugars that can be used in moderation by many families.

Cane sugar (the basis for ordinary table sugar) and, in particular, corn syrup, are *not* desirable sweetening products. None of the artificial, man-made sweeteners—such as aspartame (aka NutraSweet or Equal), sucralose (aka Splenda), or saccharine (aka Sweet'N Low)—are recommended.

If your family eats desserts and sweets daily, we recommend that you have a gluten-free, sugar-free dessert. By the way, it would be ideal to have healthier alternatives available for your child to consume as a substitute for school treats and cake at birthday parties.

Be aware that starchy carbohydrates like wheat, rice, and potatoes turn into sugar quickly in the body. Foods like pancakes, waffles, bagels, and most types of bread—even if they contain little added sugar and are gluten free—affect the body similarly to sugar. There are only a few suitable types of bread available. Most of the commercial brands, including many that are labeled "whole grain," are highly processed and refined and have a high glycemic index (meaning they turn to sugar and enter the bloodstream quickly), which is disruptive to the brain and the normal chemical processes of the body. At our clinic, we highly recommend the elimination of gluten, but if you choose to give your child gluten, true sprouted grain bread may be a better option. Unless homemade, you will probably have to purchase this bread at a health food store. Some brands to consider are Shiloh Farms and Food for Life Ezekiel 4:9.

MAKING DIETARY CHANGES

One way to introduce many of these dietary changes on behalf of your child's brain health into your family's lifestyle is to do an inventory of your household food and habits of eating. After, decide on which changes you will make immediately, and which you will do over a short period of time.

We know that habits and rituals around eating are difficult to shift, so having a plan and alternative foods in place will make the transition much smoother. Even though it will take time, the fact that you're now rethinking food, water, and nutrition options for your child and family is an awesome step. If you stay committed and consistent, you'll notice many positive things happening to you, your family, and your child over a six-month period and then beyond.

Remember, it's all about the brain and the development of your child. Once you make a shift and build these new and healthier dietary habits, your child will reap the rewards of improved bowel function, less anxiety, more attentiveness, improved behavior, better sleep, increased immune function, and a more centered home environment.

Dairy Products

Dairy products require special consideration. Like wheat, many children do not process or digest dairy easily, so you may need to reduce or eliminate these foods for a while until you can strengthen your child's digestive system. Even if your child doesn't seem to have a problem digesting dairy, the way most dairy products are now produced could trigger a sensitivity.

If your family is eating dairy, we recommend you ensure it's organic and comes from grass-fed animals. "Organic, grass-fed" milk and dairy products are the most desirable. Cows raised in the pasture eating grass, as nature intended, produce milk that is nutritionally superior to cows raised indoors and fed grain (even if that grain was organic or chemical free).

You may even choose to go a step further and purchase unpasteurized (raw) dairy products. There is much evidence that these types of milk products, when obtained from a business practicing superior farming techniques, are the most nourishing of all and the easiest to digest. (For further information on this topic, visit www.realmilk.org.)

Remember, the term "dairy" refers to all foods that are made from milk, like cheese, yogurt, sour cream, and ice cream. The milk can come from cows, goats, sheep, and buffalo. In fact, many children often tolerate goat and sheep milk more easily than cow's milk.

Healthy Fats and Oils

The body needs fats, which provide energy, protect our organs, guard us against heat loss, and aid in hormone production. Fats are also part of the myelin sheath, which insulates and protects our nerve fibers and allows them to effectively transmit impulses that affect the function of our vision, speech, movement, and thought process.

Since toxins are often stored in the fat of animals and plants, purchase fats and oils in an organic, chemical-free form. For general cooking, the most desirable ones will be solid at room temperature.

Oils and fats that provide the most health benefits include:
- Coconut oil: This is the preferred oil for cooking. It can withstand high temperatures without being damaged (which is not the case for most liquid cooking oils), and it has several health-promoting qualities.
- Palm or palm kernel oil: Desirable alternatives to use for cooking purposes. They are high in Vitamin E.
- Ghee or organic clarified butter: Safe to use for cooking and easy to make from organic butter.

Oils for low-temperature cooking:
- Cold-pressed olive oil: This can be used for very low–temperature cooking and for salad dressings.
- Butter: Organic and grass fed, if possible. Raw or unpasteurized is particularly desirable. *Note: Not recommended for children with digestive system issues or dairy sensitivities.*

Oils for room temperature use only (do not heat):
- Flaxseed oil
- Hemp oil
- Oils from nuts (walnuts, pine nuts) and seeds (pumpkin, sunflower)

You can add these oils to foods already prepared and store the bottle in the refrigerator if indicated on the label. Purchase in an *unrefined* form.

Foods containing healthy fats:
- Avocado
- Egg yolks
- Butter (especially if grass fed and unpasteurized or raw). *Not recommended for those with digestive system issues or dairy sensitivities.*
- Cream (especially if grass fed and unpasteurized or raw). *Not recommended for those with digestive system issues or dairy sensitivities.*
- Nuts and seeds (preferably raw and organic)

- "Butters" or spreads made from nuts and seeds
- Cold-water fish (especially wild Alaskan salmon, sardines, herring, and most mackerel) and caviar—these are high in very desirable omega-3 fatty acids

Try to keep a variety of these healthy fats and oils in your kitchen and include one in every meal.

Salt

High-quality, natural, and unaltered salt is another essential nutrient, because all the electrical actions of the brain and the body require sodium, found in salt. Salt balances body fluid and ensures that your nerves and muscles are performing at their most efficient and effective. It is also necessary for transmitting electrical signals through the body. Salt also helps the body to absorb vitamins and minerals, balance electrolytes, and maintain acid/alkaline balance.

You may be thinking, *But isn't salt bad for you?* We're not talking about the standard white table salt you find in diners or on your kitchen table because that type of salt has been stripped of natural elements except for sodium chloride. It also contains artificial agents that reduce clumping. Regular use of table salt can cause acidic edema, cellulite, and lead to high blood pressure and cardiovascular disease. It can even affect the body's vitamin D levels.

We recommend replacing all the white salt in your kitchen with a natural, whole salt like Celtic or French (Sel Marin de Guerande) sea salt or Himalayan pink salt—these all contain as many as eighty-five elemental minerals. Himalayan salt, in particular, has risen in popularity, making it easy to find in most grocery stores. Be sure to buy one that is authentic (sourced from the Himalayas of northern Pakistan)—it will be pink in color.

You can also buy a larger quantity of the somewhat coarse, "light gray" Celtic salt (which is less expensive than the others) to be used for general cooking purposes. Since this is moist and does not contain anti-caking agents, keeping it in a small dish on your kitchen counter is a convenient way to use it.

For the table, you might want to purchase the "fine ground" Celtic salt in a shaker jar plus an additional bag to use for refills. This salt is also moist but is slightly finer and therefore can be used in a shaker with larger holes.

FOOD SENSITIVITIES

Food sensitivities or intolerances are increasingly common today, in both children and adults. The past decade has seen a surge in the number of people who require or desire a gluten-free diet.

Gluten is a protein molecule found in many grains and processed/refined foods, as well as in various hair-care products, Play-Doh, and glues. It's most prominent in wheat, which is the main ingredient in bread and pasta, two food items that kids typically love. Many children find it difficult to digest or break down gluten, triggering allergies and an array of troublesome side effects and gut-health problems like constipation and irritable bowel syndrome. The consumption of gluten adversely affects brain function (the brain gets foggy and irritated) in many children with special needs we see.

Thankfully, there's now an abundance of gluten-free items stocked on supermarket shelves, allowing you and your children to enjoy pasta, breakfast cereal, bread, and snacks. However, we do not recommend these with every meal, as they are still processed and refined substances and not the ideal whole, real foods we're aiming for.

Casein is a protein found in milk and milk products. Its molecular structure is similar to gluten, and it's also hard to digest. Like gluten, it can lead to intestinal and neurological problems. Casein has also been known to cause recurrent ear infections, allergies, upper-respiratory infections, and skin rashes. If you notice that your child has any of these conditions, you will want to eliminate dairy for at least three months and see if that alleviates the problem. Clinically, we notice that children are healthier when they are gluten free and primarily dairy free. As with gluten free, there are also many options and milk substitutes available, but—and it is a big but—they are not always healthy. The healthiest milk substitutes are coconut milk or milks made from water blended with organic, raw nuts and seeds. There are wonderful healthy beverage recipes online that you can make at home, which will offer a wonderful alternative to milk.

Gluten, dairy, corn, and soy are at the top of the list of foods most likely to cause a variety of problems in the brain and body, and many children, as well as parents, may benefit from removing them entirely from the diet.

DIGESTIVE SYSTEM FUNCTIONING

The medical community considers the gut as the "second brain"—this is actually the enteric nervous system—so, not surprisingly, gut health goes hand and hand with nutrition.

The gut pathway goes from the mouth all the way down through the esophagus to the stomach, the small intestine, large intestine, and all the way out through the colon—it includes the whole digestive system. And if something happens to you or there is stress in your life, where do you feel that stress? In the gut, right? That's because your vagus nerve runs straight from your brain stem into your lungs, heart, and stomach. In fact, when you "go with your gut" or have a "gut feeling" about something, you are using your brain via the vagus nerve. That's why it's necessary to keep our guts healthy and our stress levels down. As the gut goes, so does the brain, so having optimum digestive and gut health is a significant factor in brain health and development.

Overall, we manufacture more than 50 percent of our neurotransmitters in our large intestines, and more than 95 percent of serotonin (the "happy brain" chemical) is produced in the intestines. Think of our large intestines as an elegant compost pile supplying wonderful neurotransmitters to the brain while it also effectively and efficiently releases waste and toxins.

One other important fact about the digestive system: it's very closely linked with the immune and nervous systems. There are more immune cells located in our intestinal lining than in any other location in the body. When digestive system health is improved, improvement is made in the immune and nervous systems, too.

Many children have less than optimal digestive system functioning, but parents are often unaware of it. If your child has reflux or vomiting, excessive burping or flatulence (gas), frequent stomachaches, bowel movements that are not formed or not daily or especially smelly, food sensitivities, or constipation, then their digestive system might not be working correctly. If your child has difficulty sleeping, paying attention, has skin/hair/nail problems, or is unusually irritable or angry, these may also be signs of digestive system problems.

Digestion—the breaking down of food into particles small enough to be absorbed and then utilized by the body—is the job of the top section of the digestive tract. Elimination is the job of the lower section. Good, daily elimination is vital for all of us. Bowel movements three or four times a day are not problematic, if they are not watery or diarrhea. A healthy bowel movement is usually formed like a sausage or banana, soft, not especially smelly, is without undigested food particles, and is not slimy or greasy.

Regardless of the specifics of the diet you choose to give your child, a tailored and consistent regimen is recommended, as is one that restricts or altogether eliminates problematic or difficult-to-digest foods. Digestive enzymes, probiotics, and prebiotics (or prebiotic foods, such as chicory, leek, and onion) are particularly helpful in restoring optimal functioning to the digestive system.

Again, the human body needs high-quality nutrients to be delivered to all its cells daily, particularly in a growing child. The body also produces naturally a variety of waste products and toxins that need to be eliminated daily. Some of this waste material is produced by the cells themselves during their normal functioning. Some waste materials or toxins enter the body from the outside through food, water, air, and our skin. The body has specific detoxifying chemical pathways to deal with these various toxins. Our clinical experience suggests these pathways do not function as well as they should when a child is neurologically compromised.

Detoxification is handled primarily by the liver and the kidneys. The toxins processed by the liver are dumped into the top of the intestines and eliminated through the lower intestines through bowel movements. Toxins handled by the kidneys are flushed out by the urine that is produced by the kidneys. The body also eliminates unwanted substances through the lungs (with exhalation) and the skin (by sweating). Of all these avenues of elimination, the liver and the colon (lower intestine) handle the most substantial amount of waste material. That is why constipation (anything less than complete, daily elimination in our opinion) is so undesirable.

Transit time from the mouth to the colon should take about one day. The longer it takes the body to eliminate waste in the form of a bowel movement, the more likely it is that the child will become constipated, and that will bring toxicity to the entire system.

To help prevent constipation, ensure that your child has:

- Adequate daily water intake (ounces equal to half your child's weight, as explained earlier). So if your child is 80 pounds, 30 to 40 oz of water per day would be ideal.
- Adequate daily fiber. Vegetables, fruits, legumes (properly prepared), gluten-free whole grains, nuts, and seeds are naturally high in fiber. Some children may benefit from a fiber supplement. Start with one-half the recommended amount stated on the label, along with adequate water.
- Probiotic (beneficial bacteria) supplementation through food and supplements.
- Cooked, dark-green, leafy vegetables (one to two daily servings).
- Exercise and movement.
- A comprehensive digestive enzyme with each meal.

If your child is following the recommended dietary and supplemental program, as well as the previous guidelines, and is still experiencing constipation, you need to delve even deeper into their diet to determine if there are any food allergies or environmental sensitivities. You should also consider consulting with a holistic gastroenterologist, naturopath, homeopath, chiropractor, cranial-sacral therapist, lymph drainage therapist, fascia therapist, or an acupuncturist.

If your child is experiencing indigestion, bloating, or excessive gas, an old-fashioned remedy using raw (unpasteurized, unfiltered) apple cider vinegar can be very helpful. Purchase this item at a natural food store and mix one teaspoon (5 ml) in a glass of water. Have your child sip this water at mealtimes, after mealtimes, or throughout the day. You should also have them drink or rinse out their mouth with plain water, so the acidity of the vinegar doesn't irritate the mouth or teeth. Using a straw to sip the drink can also be helpful.

Food combining is another technique that aids in digestion and digestive system health. If your child has problems, this can be a beneficial way to eat. The main guidelines for food combining are:

- Fruit should be eaten alone and before or well after mealtimes. If your child can eat yogurt or nuts/seeds or butter made from them, these foods also can combine well with fruit.
- Animal protein and starchy carbohydrates ("fast carbs") should not be eaten at the same meal. This can require quite a change in eating habits but can also be very effective. Non-starchy carbohydrates and good fats combine well with both animal protein and starchy carbs. If your child is following food-combining principles, we suggest that breakfast and lunch be comprised of animal protein.

NUTRITIONAL SUPPLEMENTS

In our many years of clinical experience, depending on the child's neurology and digestive functioning, we have found nutritional supplements to be extremely helpful. However, it's important to remember that supplements are just that. A whole-food, nourishing diet is foundational and most important. The supplements—whether vitamins, minerals, oils, other nutrients, and digestive system aids—will enhance that diet and the normal processes of the body.

If you think that supplements will be helpful, find a qualified nutrition expert to work with.

When using nutritional supplements, here are some basic rules to follow:

- Follow the label's instructions about proper storage. In general, most oils and probiotics are best kept refrigerated.
- Supplements should be kept out of sunlight and away from direct heat. Discard any cotton inside a bottle once you open it.
- Keep lids screwed on tightly and keep bottles away from small children.
- As with food and many other things in life, there can be a disparity in the quality of the supplemental products. The basic ingredients, filler materials, processing, and storage are all important. You can visit www.healthbasics.net to locate high-quality products at reasonable prices.
- If your child is new to supplementation with quality products, please introduce them slowly—one at a time. Start with one-half of the recommended amounts for the first week, and then increase to the full amount. If your child is particularly sensitive, one-quarter of the recommended dosage may be more appropriate for the first week, one-half for the second week, three-quarters for the third week, and then the full recommended amount. Introduce one product at a time, at weekly intervals.

EXERCISE

As noted in chapter six, ontogenetic exercise is perfect for your child. Crawling to develop the pons, creeping on hands and knees to develop the midbrain, walking and running for the cortex, and gymnastics to develop the cerebellum—these are ideal ways to exercise and get organized at the same time. We encourage following the earlier recommendations and integrating these types of activities into your child's day. Pursue what your child will enjoy most, whether bicycle riding, horseback riding, swimming, jumping rope, or playing sports.

SLEEP

Having a good night's sleep is critical to everyone's health. Sleep supplies energy. It fosters development, recharges the body and the brain, and promotes learning, relaxation, and improved behavior. Sleep problems are commonplace among most children, but even more so when a child is neurologically compromised. Most have difficulty falling asleep and staying asleep.

According to the National Sleep Foundation, the amount of sleep that children need varies with age, but these are the basic guidelines:

AGE OF CHILD	HOURS OF SLEEP
NEWBORNS (0–3 MONTHS)	14 to 17 hours
INFANTS (4–11 MONTHS)	12 to 15 hours
TODDLERS (1–2 YEARS)	11 to 14 hours
PRESCHOOLERS (3–5 YEARS)	10 to 13 hours
SCHOOL-AGED CHILDREN (6–13 YEARS)	9 to 11 hours
TEENAGERS (14–17 YEARS)	8 to 10 hours

Knowing the approximate hours of sleep required for your child will help you to set their bedtime and wake-up time appropriately. A good way to determine how much sleep is needed is to pick a day when your child can get to bed before ten at night at the latest, and then let them sleep until they wake on their own without an alarm, the sun in their face, or other stimuli. Then count the number of hours slept. In the absence of a sleep disorder or multiple awakenings during the night, this is the number of hours your child's body and brain need at this time for optimal rejuvenation.

Create an environment conducive to sleeping. Your child will obtain the highest quality rest in his own bed, in a darkened, quiet bedroom that is cool. The mattress should be very firm. The bedding and sleepwear should be a breathable fabric like cotton or bamboo. One to two hours before bedtime should be a calming-down period, without exposure to screens: no television, electronics, or video games. Warm baths before bedtime can also be sleep inducing.

We encourage establishing a structured bedtime routine. For example, a bath followed by story time and a good night prayer and kiss. Some children who find it challenging downregulating—quieting or calming down on their own—can also benefit from quiet music, nature sounds, or aromatherapy diffused into the room. Whatever routine you create, follow the same regimen every night, as this will become comforting to your child and eventually enhance the quality of his sleep. If someone else puts the child to bed—an older sibling, Grandma, or the babysitter—please ensure that they become familiar with and follow the routine you established.

Many brain-injured children have difficulty understanding routine, so to assist in the acclimation process, you might consider creating a picture book that illustrates your nightly routine. You can take and add in photos that depict bath time, pajamas, reading a bedtime story, the child's bedroom at night, etc., so that the routine becomes an illustrated story. This is a helpful tool that you or anyone else minding your child at night can use to help ease your child through the bedtime routine.

ENVIRONMENT

There are many aspects to creating a healthy environment. At a minimum, your home should be clean, tidy, and devoid of toxins.

Creating a clean environment is conducive to growth, health, and learning. When you have a child with special needs at home, there's not always the time or energy to be perfectly organized—we understand that. But doing the best you can to improve the environment will make you and your family feel better in many ways. Take things one step at a time.

Keep your home clean. Most of us are keenly aware that a clean, toxic-free environment is beneficial for your child, so a little effort goes a long way. As you are most likely very busy doing the big things, if you can afford it, consider hiring a professional house cleaner and supply them with organic cleaning products. If not, do your best to tidy up when you can and clean one room of your house each day or every other day. It would be fantastic to have everyone involved in a Saturday morning team cleanup, too!

Remember to check bathrooms, kitchens, basements, and garages for any signs of mold and mildew and address these problems immediately to avoid triggering allergies or the onset of a respiratory issue. Cleaning—and using the right cleaning products—will help to remove any potential toxins in your home.

Take stock of cleaning and personal-care products. As mentioned previously, we highly recommend switching out your personal care and cleaning products with those that are more organic and natural, so that you can avoid harsh chemicals and fragrances. Many children with special needs are very sensitive to scents, so we recommend using only "fragrance-free" organic products.

Most household cleaners, as well as laundry detergents, are filled with chemicals that can be inhaled or absorbed through the skin when used. They can also permeate the air in your home. Many cleansers, sprays, carpet cleaners, and air fresheners contain chemicals linked to asthma and cancer, and children are more vulnerable to the effects of these products than adults. If you have pets, they are also vulnerable.

You can replace these cleaning supplies with a spray bottle of equal parts white vinegar and water. Even in the yard, where the kids roll around and play, you can purchase natural gardening and lawn products and feel good about completing the circuit of cleaning inside and outside the house for your children.

Finally, consider scents you use on yourself. If you wear perfume or cologne, purchase fragrances and oils that are organic or made from all-natural ingredients. You and your partner can still smell fresh and nice by making your own scents using essential oils. Once you try this, you will never go back to using anything else.

Cut down on EMF pollution. Electromagnetic fields—EMFs for short—are invisible frequencies generated by electrical appliances and electronic devices. Many children and some adults are acutely sensitive to this type of pollution. These are challenging to avoid, because we live in an electronic world filled with TVs, tablets, computers, microwave ovens, cell phones, Wi-Fi signals, and even fluorescent light bulbs. The best you can do is limit your child's direct exposure to them. You can reduce EMF exposure by turning off Wi-Fi when not in use, using special computer screen covers and laptop pads, and holding cell phones and tablets away from your body. Limit TV time and, when you do watch TV together, don't let children sit too close to the TV screen. In 1996, the World Health Organization established the International EMF Project to assess both health and environmental effects of EMFs. You can learn more about their studies at www.who.int/peh-emf/en.

IMPACT OF ELECTRONICS AND SCREEN TIME

Besides the potential risks of EMFs, electronic devices have other detrimental effects on children and parents. Personal connection is being compromised more than ever before. Walk down any street, and most of the people coming in your direction are busy with their phones. When we travel through airports, we see it all the time: kids are playing on their cell phones and no one is talking. If we went back in time thirty years and everyone was reading a book, we might think that was ideal. The thing is, electronics are more addictive for the brain than books. The lights, dings, superfast information, and games make it difficult to disengage. If you've ever seen the challenges some children face neurologically when trying to disengage from a TV, tablet, phone, or computer game, this is even more reason to sprint toward creating a healthier balance. We all are susceptible to being distracted and preoccupied with the urgency of knowing everything right now and responding to incoming information. By setting personal boundaries and making time to put technology on pause, we can reconnect 100 percent with our kids and become more tuned in to the hurt child.

We understand that electronics keep children occupied and safe when parents need a quick break or to help occupy a child while at a restaurant. But overall, it would be ideal to gradually diminish screen time since it unbalances the limbic brain.

From the earliest months of life, children nowadays are hyperstimulated by toys that use sound effects and bright lights. Some companies with educational missions support the exposure of our children to electronics—from devices that dangle a tablet above a sleeping child's crib to potty-training seats with an iPad that encourages toddlers to distract themselves while learning an essential biological function.

This trend may be having an adverse effect. A recent study by TARGet Kids! (www.targetkids.ca/publications), a practice-based research network in Toronto, revealed that the more time children between the ages of six months and two years spent using handheld screens, the more likely they were to experience speech delays.

Increased screen time has been linked to ADHD, sleep difficulties, childhood obesity, behavior problems, and decreased academic performance, as well as delays in developing social skills.

To remedy this, start by setting an example. Children mimic adult behavior, so be conscious of the time you spend on your devices when you are with your child and curtail using them. When you're together as a family, put away electronic devices during dinner or other family meals and gatherings. Limit your child's computer and TV time. Replace screen time with other activities. Take a walk or go for a drive. Go to the park. Play a board game or read a book together. Most importantly, reconnect. That stimulates the limbic system. Read facial expressions and give your child time to do the same. (Remember: it takes children on the spectrum and those with Down syndrome even longer to process whatever emotion you are displaying.) When addressing your child, pause after each facial interaction so he can learn what every expression means. Try to play games that are appropriate for your child's neurological age. Most of all, spend time together to practice and work out how to interact. Even being together during moments of quiet and boredom are helpful.

Any type of "together time" is crucial. Shifting away from electronics to interpersonal experiences will improve your child's ability to socialize and to obtain and process information that will have a positive impact on brain development.

PEOPLE

Family members and friends also have an influence on your child's health. That influence can be positive or questionable, or sometimes both. Awareness and mindfulness are critical here. We collect energy from people, so if you are surrounded by people who are happy and energetic problem solvers, and who talk about positive things, you're going to acquire good energy from them. On the other side, having people around who are negative—those who shout, complain, criticize, give up, or bully—is detrimental to your and your child's well-being.

Sometimes friends and family members are oblivious to the impact their words or behaviors have on your child. If someone uses language in an inappropriate manner in the presence of your child, take them aside and speak with them privately about your concerns. If you point things out, most family members and friends will understand and take measures to change their behavior.

When people are cheerful, warm, friendly, and interested, you see the positive influence on your child. Children are sensitive and know when someone is sincere and authentic. If you notice your child's face light up when a particular person comes into the room, take note. Pay attention to who makes your child laugh or who calms her down. These are the people you will want to have in your home—whom you also might consider recruiting to become part of your support team.

Before visitors come to your house, perhaps think about sharing some of your "house rules" with them in advance, particularly if you anticipate that they will interact with your child. Such rules can include bringing your child something other than candy, cupcakes, or sweets.

Prepare your children for visitors *ahead* of their arrival. You may find it helpful to show them pictures of who will arrive, when they will arrive, why they are coming to visit, and when they will be leaving. You have all this information in your head naturally, so you are proactive and secure. However, hurt children can get confused and disoriented around visitors in their home, and may act unsociably because they do not understand the parameters of the visit. Even if Grandma and Grandpa are coming over, it is helpful to communicate and prepare your child for their arrival in advance. You can make a note of the visit on the family whiteboard or scroll through photos of the grandparents on your phone with your child so she will recognize them when they arrive.

While sufficient quiet and rest are vital to overall health, so is a bountiful supply of laughter and enjoyment (this applies to you, too!). We know it is a challenge, but whenever possible, please try not to be so caught up in the seriousness and intensity of your child's care or program that you neglect the chance to have a good belly laugh together from time to time. Laughter is always the best medicine.

Finally, treasured family members and friends bring joy and love. Surrounding your child with those who love her unconditionally, and who understand and support the boundaries you have in place, will bring happiness to your child's life. If your child cannot respond to touch or is not comfortable being touched, there are neurological reasons for this. Give him or her space and time to acclimate, and have family members demonstrate their affection through language expressed from the heart with tenderness. In time, your child's comfort level will grow and the bonding reflex, limbic brain, and sense of tactile sensation will be restored.

FAMILY SUCCESS STORY

I will admit that as an acupuncturist who has spent a ton of time studying nutrition, I didn't expect to learn much from the nutrition program. When I brought my son, Remy, to the Family Hope Center, I already knew how important diet was. As a child with an impressively rare genetic disorder that causes epilepsy, global delays, and a long list of challenges, Remy was already on a diet full of whole, organic foods, and void of gluten or dairy to avoid inflammation or leaky gut.

I had read about using the keto diet for epilepsy, but as a single mom who was already juggling quite a lot, I was daunted by the prospect of measuring and weighing food. Instead of putting Remy on a strict ketogenic diet, we worked with the Family Hope Center team to reduce grains and sugar, both of which increase his tremor and can trigger seizures. By looking more closely at Remy's diet and what we were eating, I was able to find ways to make easy substitutions and ensure he was getting the right nutrients and the right fats to support his development. The team helped me work smarter, not harder.

Instead of cooking with olive oil, which goes rancid when it's heated, we switched to ghee and coconut oil. Instead of two to three fruits a day, we cut that down and added more nuts and seeds. Increasing Remy's water intake and decreasing the coconut water I gave him drastically reduced the amount of sugar he was getting. And those coconut yogurts he loved—eighteen grams of sugar per serving! I switched those to sugar free and added CMT and chia or hemp seeds to them.

By making simple changes in both our diets, we were able to see pretty remarkable changes in Remy very quickly. His muscle tone is significantly better and he's now beginning to walk independently. His tremor is almost gone and now he only has seizures when he's sick. Remy is now able to engage with toys and other children more meaningfully. It's amazing to watch him interact more with the world around him. I love watching him notice new things. His neurological age doubled from our first session to our second session at Family Hope Center, and honestly, I was doing less work with him than I had been before!

While I was already fortunate enough to know how important whole foods are, the Family Hope Center helped me isolate the ways that I could fine-tune the hard work I was doing. What has been incredible is the difference in both of us. Remy and I both have more energy and focus and continue to feel better and better. Good food really is the best form of medicine, and when done right, it can heal the whole family!

—*Chloe, Remy's mom*

NEURO-PARENTING POINTS

- Children with special needs have unique sensitivities to food, their environment, and anything related to the five senses. Even minor changes can affect a child's emotions and health.
- Optimum health is achieved by the body's ability to collect and distribute energy successfully. The sources through which we gather that energy include:
  - Air
  - Water
  - Food

- Exercise
- Sleep
- Environment
- People

- These seven sources of energy can be either nutritious or toxic depending on their level of quality. Strive to provide your child with a safe, clean, and nurturing environment, so that he has the proper energy to thrive.
- When it comes to your child's well-being, take measures to:
  - Filter the air in the house through an air purifier, house-plants, and HEPA filters.
  - Spend time outdoors in the fresh air and natural sunlight.
  - Provide pure water for drinking.
  - Prepare and serve organic whole foods—avoid processed and packaged food.
  - Avoid gluten, casein, sugar, and food additives.
  - Use excellent quality salt.
  - Use healthy fats and oils when cooking.
  - Include exercise in the daily routine.
  - Create a structured sleep routine—sleep is vital for energy and development.
  - Keep the home clean using toxin-free products.
  - Cut down on EMF pollution.

- Expose your child to people who are friendly, warm, and positive, who will provide unconditional love and support.

CHAPTER 8

GROWING AND CARING
FOR YOURSELF

Reading up to this point, we hope you've developed a more thorough understanding of the brain, the importance of nutrition, what tools you can use to stimulate healthy brain development, and how to measure your child's progress over time. An equally important and often overlooked piece of the healing equation is how to incorporate yourself in a plan toward wellness, and how to take care of your own needs.

We've worked alongside parents and caregivers for almost forty years. Again and again we've seen the relentless internal drive of parents who want to do everything they can to help their children. We've seen it within ourselves. We know how hard it is, and how much you have to sacrifice. When you personally have a child with special needs, it's difficult to explain the extraordinary amount of work and real, not imagined, stress that devours your day-to-day life.

Hyperfocus is needed to support your child and keep the family aloft. However, the cost of this focus usually comes with a pace that's simply not sustainable long term. When a parent is navigating their hurt child through developmental and physiological hurdles, operating by definition in crisis mode, self-care is most typically the first thing to fall by the wayside. This is normal.

The pace is maddening. The demands on your time aren't sustainable. How do we find a balance? How can we all thrive in the family? How do we move from parenting in sprint mode to finding ways to successfully move into marathon mode, a direction that's imperative to reach for the whole family to thrive?

Wherever you are in your journey, our hope is that you see the possibility for change in your future. It doesn't matter if you're currently navigating overwhelming challenges combined with feelings of sadness and grief, or just feeling out of balance and wanting a little more personal time. The possibility for change is there, in time.

We also hope you give yourself permission to heal alongside your partner and family and seek the necessary support, compassion, and understanding all of us need. In this pivotal chapter we want to walk beside you wherever you are in this process. We want to help guide you by sharing what we've seen and experienced as medical professionals and parents. Ultimately, we hope you'll find some practical skills and ideas and take away a tool or even a toolbox to help you take one small step at a time in the direction of looking after yourselves and bringing hope and confidence back into your life.

COMMON FEELINGS AND THOUGHTS

What's obvious, and should almost go without saying, is the reality of how parenting automatically shifts your attention and affects both you and your relationships. It's not something we can be fully ready for ahead of time. Like many parents, as a mother, I (Carol) didn't feel 100 percent ready to take on parenting, and when my first child decided to arrive three weeks early, I was amazed at how I rapidly moved into a combination of feeling out of control and yet super focused. Matthew and I are very different but complementary people. I like to have time to think about things, be prepared, and plan ahead. This early birth made it necessary to race to the hospital before I even had time to pack a bag with a change of clothes for myself and my baby!

Once that baby arrived, though, I had no choice but to embrace this newness. I was surprised by the overwhelming feeling of being responsible for a life. Even though I had a great deal of experience in childcare and education, my limbic brain produced this overwhelming, hyperfocused feeling. Now it was real. Now it was personal.

Doctors, midwives, and parenting books often prepare mothers for pregnancy and the birth of their baby. However, there's very little preparation for what comes next, and support from friends, family, and doctors often fades after the first few weeks. Parents are left to navigate the unexpected, and to often balance feelings of confusion and uncertainty with their own high expectations for their performance as a parent. When a child is born with a health issue or experiences a debilitating illness or trauma, that processing of feelings can quickly and easily lend itself to self-blame.

Parents often find themselves at a loss for whom to turn to for advice. Or, conversely, they're often overwhelmed with advice to sort out. A family struggling to find support for a child with a rare condition may not know anyone else who can empathize with their situation. While family and friends can assist with advice on raising a typical newborn, it can be incredibly isolating to be the only person you know working to support a child who isn't well. When an injury or illness occurs, or development doesn't have the expected outcome, additional feelings of guilt, grief, loss, and even trauma are part of the process. This is normal. Recognizing the presence of these feelings and seeing them for what they are is key.

For instance, grieving over the lost dream of a healthy child can manifest as self-blame and doubt in one's ability to function adequately as a parent. Mothers and fathers in this situation will often stumble with guilt, asking themselves questions such as: "Did I do something wrong when I was pregnant?" or "Is there something I could have done differently since he/she was born?"

Watch out for faulty assumptions. They're easy to make as a parent. Thoughts like *I must not be a good enough teacher, or my child would be learning*; or *My child behaves this way because I'm not a good enough disciplinarian/coach*;

or *I am just not smart enough or well equipped to help this child*, will come over you. But they don't have to *control* you.

Many parents who have faced a difficult birth or suddenly find themselves caring for a child with a debilitating illness or injury become hyperfocused on their child's health. They overlook the trauma they experienced themselves as a result of these events. In fact, many parents have their own trauma attached to a difficult birth or an illness or injury that put them in the hospital with their child. Not to mention the compounding effect of repeated hospitalizations due to illnesses, recurring seizures, or frequent follow-up and testing visits. Parents find themselves reliving the trauma and fear along with their child during these repeat events.

Remember to breathe and clear your head for a minute. It's hard, but it can be done. Our brains are designed to hyperfocus on survival during times of crisis. A traumatic experience, such as learning that your child is diagnosed with a debilitating illness or injury, can instantly initiate this response in caregivers, as humans are neurologically programmed to engage either a "fight," "flight," or "freeze" response when faced with danger. The brain has a difficult time distinguishing the level of danger your child is in and often automatically goes to DEFCON 4! Harm to your child's body or brain will activate you to respond as if to a personal threat. You may start feeling overly vigilant, struggle to sleep, feel constant pressure to keep up productive output (the "fight" response), or feel paralyzed (the "freeze" response) after receiving an unexpected or even an expected diagnosis.

Small bursts of productive energy can help navigate a time of crisis. Eventually a child will no longer need their parents to be in crisis mode, though. When that happens, the expected relief can be hard to find, as it's difficult for a parent to downshift and let go of the feelings attached to hyperactivated states. Trauma will automatically shift our brain stem and limbic brain.

Therefore, understanding where you and your spouse are in the timeline of this journey is the first step toward healing for yourself. In our experience, all parents of hurt children arrive at a crossroads: *I can stay where I am and manage this. Or can I find a path that will lead me toward the healthiest version of my family and myself?* If the road you take is the latter, start by asking what small changes you can make today to help yourself and your family thrive.

PRACTICAL STEPS TO MOVE TOWARD CARING FOR YOURSELF

Unfortunately, the quick fix of "putting a lid on your emotions" isn't realistic. Turn your brain-based approach inward: Acknowledge any thoughts or feelings you are having and evaluate their root cause. Emotions are thought of as originating in our limbic brain. Emotional knowledge in the more primitive areas of our brain can feel overwhelming and nebulous. Help yourself to better understand your feelings by speaking them aloud and thus bringing them into the frontal cortex, which houses the verbal centers of our brain. You might verbalize to yourself, "I feel sad because my child has seizures." This acknowledges the reality of the sadness and loss you feel. Next, say, "I am thankful that I have knowledge to change my child's diet, which can help their brain develop and reduce these seizures." Finally, connect this emotional processing to the impulse to help by preparing some healthy food for your child. Helping yourself regain balance with this proactive strategy can allow you to dedicate a better, healthier version of yourself to the task of helping your hurt child.

Be aware that the guilt, disappointment, and sadness you feel will all but certainly come back in waves, often at times you least expect it. Cultivating a mindset and countering this by moving through with intentionality is key. The process is one of gradually moving forward. Being the parent of a hurt child isn't a role you asked for. Over time, when you look back, your strength and your ability to wisely care for both your family and yourself while facing these difficult times will refresh you and remind you that you're a superhero.

Gradually allow yourself to let go of the undeserved blame you feel. Remember, holding on to fear can become a coping mechanism for parents who have received traumatic news about their child. It can be difficult to allow yourself to relax when you're worried that disaster will strike again. We call this hypervigilance. Face the reality of the problem while remembering you did *nothing* wrong. *This is a problem in my child's brain, and I am putting a plan in place to support their growth and development.*

When we weren't seeing our own child make progress, we were often tempted to believe it must have been because of our own lack of effort or skill. A gentler and more solution-focused approach would have been to see the brain dysfunction for what it was and to be patient with ourselves and the child. We had to remind ourselves: "It's not about you, it's not about her—it's about her brain." Keeping myself focused on executing our plan helped ensure consistency and a much healthier outlook for everyone in our family.

Parents of children with special needs, whatever the degree and extent, find they must become extraordinary in their ability to be organized, stronger, more energetic, and more focused for their child. If only we could develop the necessary superpowers overnight! But that's not how it goes, and it's never healthy to blame the self for not perfectly and immediately living up to those extremely high standards.

It's critical to master the challenging task of remaining patient with the process you're going through. As parents, you are the solution to your child's problems. Being realistic yet optimistic, and staying within the brain while keeping your emotions healthy, will move you toward your goals.

BALANCE

Ask the question: How do I maintain balance for myself and my family? I want to have healthy expectations, increase my energy, and not allow my feelings to constantly deplete that energy.

Taking and finding time for yourself is the first step toward achieving this balance. Getting to the place where you can have healthy expectations takes awareness and attention, though. It's a process that requires you to be patient with yourself as you go through this journey.

To start, do you know where you are in this journey? You may be feeling stuck. Perhaps just getting through your day is all you can think about. Maybe you just feel a little unbalanced but are ready to think about putting some attention on yourself. No matter where you are, the importance of looking after yourself requires attention. This is ultimately your journey as parents, and you need to decide what to do to look after yourself and your family.

POTENTIAL OBSTACLES AND FINDING SOLUTIONS

Studies show the birth of a new child, on average, adds about twenty-four hours to the workweek of the typical parent. Now consider how much extra time and care a child with special needs requires. The reality is that an overwhelmed, burned-out parent has fewer resources to give to their child. It's critical to evaluate whether it's sustainable to continue to meet the challenges you're facing as you have been, or whether it's time to ask for help.

Parents operating in superhero mode may find it difficult to ask for assistance. Asking for help can feel like admitting you're not able to fully support your child. Thinking you can do it all alone simply isn't realistic. Recognize when you're feeling burned out by periodically evaluating yourself, as you do for your child. Give yourself permission to ask for assistance, so that you can be the strongest, healthiest version of yourself. Both you and your child deserve it!

NUTRITION AND MEALS

Eat healthy. As a family. The recommendations in chapter seven can be followed for the entire family. This can put everyone on a path toward ultimate health and well-being, and it can make life easier, as it's much more convenient and practical to cook just one meal for the whole household. If you try to accommodate each person's tastes, you will potentially find yourself cooking several different meals. This just isn't sustainable.

Lead by example! A child requiring a special diet will feel more included if they see the whole family eating the same foods they are. Demonstrate your commitment to health through the foods you choose to put on your table. Once you start eating this way, you'll find the cravings for things like simple carbs will diminish.

We do tend to have an emotional attachment to our food, so some foods will be difficult to let go of. When stressed, we often gravitate to foods that emotionally feel good in the moment, but too often that food is not what our bodies and brains need.

Be honest with yourself about your habits or tendencies. First, adjust for health by taking out foods that you know are unhealthy and replacing them. Next, look at the things you do for comfort. Certainly, comfort eating/drinking can be a good thing, but can you also make it healthy? Can you replace snuggling on the couch with a hot chocolate for a nice warm cup of herbal tea? Trust me, your brain will be happier!

Maybe you really want to have a family meal together, but it just isn't working because of disruptions, distractions, or the effort you need to spend focusing on your child with special needs. If this is the case, you could feed your child first, and then he can sit to join the family for the social aspect of the mealtime, and this way he is not as disruptive. Maybe you want to eat as a couple as many of our families do; they find that feeding their child early and then putting them to bed gives them the ability to eat in peace and enjoy some time for themselves and each other. This makes a lot of sense.

SLEEP

One of the main roles of sleeping is to restore and heal the brain.

I know of fathers and mothers who sit up all night holding their child in a chair or staying with them on the couch because it's the only place their child sleeps. However, the parent then suffers. It is not unusual for a child to need a parent to regulate them in order to fall asleep and stay asleep. Some children prefer one parent over another to regulate them, which again creates an imbalance in the home.

Ideally, the child needs to be able to learn to regulate themselves and sleep without relying on someone else. However, this can take time and may require some outside help. It is our advice to work patiently but directly to establish a healthy sleep routine for your child because you both need your sleep!

To be a healthy adult, our brains and bodies need seven to eight hours of sleep. Many of the parents we've seen over the years are getting significantly less. In fact, they're often lucky to get three to four hours of uninterrupted sleep—and this just isn't enough or sustainable for the long haul. If you are sleep deprived because you are up and down with your child, please find healthy ways to get sleep, and it should be one of your top priorities. We have sleep guidelines in chapter seven, and the overall nutritional changes could be just what your child needs. We have seen parents applying these changes, and within a few weeks, they and their child are beginning to achieve better sleep. Having the improved bedtime routine helps with the downregulation and the ability to ease into sleep and stay asleep.

If sleep time is a major struggle to master, we recommend you get help and support. The first option would be to switch off between parents, sharing the night shift. Or you could split the night shift with one parent going to bed early while one stays in bed later. If you're not able to quickly move into a routine, ask and accept help from outside family members, friends, or a respite center. Some parents have a helper take over some of the night shifts so they can sleep in peace. Another alternative when you don't have help is to sleep when your child sleeps during the day. Put off the house chores for now and get some sleep! Give yourself permission to sleep!

ROUTINES

We like patterns and routines. They're good for our brains. Your child will work well with a routine, and it will benefit you also. Babies' and young children's routines are ever changing as they develop. This can be challenging for parents as they begin to feel like they have just settled into a reasonable routine when the child changes by dropping a nap or needing multiple extended feeding times. We must be on our toes to readjust again and again to our hurt child while maintaining some structure with the rest of the family. This takes wisdom as it is difficult to be constantly one step ahead of the routines necessary for a sane household.

Children with special needs by definition of the injury struggle to follow or get in the flow of routines due to disorganization in their brain. Sleep challenges, illnesses, seizure, and the list goes on—all are disruptive. It is important and doable to create a balanced routine and by establishing great consistency guide your child's eating and sleeping into a healthy pattern. Do not feel bad about creating this clear structure—the brain of the child is desperate for it.

Meanwhile, there is you. While you may need to focus on your child's routine for a time, don't wait too long to establish your own healthy routine—get up at a set time, work out, establish quiet time, take your shower, and dress for the day. It sounds funny, but try to avoid staying in your pj's all day. You will feel so much better for it!

YOUR STATE OF MIND

Do you find you feel trapped by your circumstances but also your inability to stay positive? You're not alone. And you're not going crazy. Acknowledge your thoughts. They are real. They are based on true fear and concern for your child and their future. Tell yourself, "Yes, this is sad, but I have solutions and things to do." Be gentle with yourself when redirecting your negative thoughts. Take time to acknowledge that it hurts you to see your child suffering. You can replace those thoughts with actions for your child and family. When we do things, we move out of our limbic brain (feelings) and into our cortex (thinking and action). Being in the present for both you and your child is the healthiest place. It does require some work and practice to learn to process the guilt and emotions and move forward into action. And to do it with joy! We have seen the most joy from parents when they are able to celebrate the little victories. Take time to acknowledge how far you have come, how much you have learned, and the great changes that you have made to your lifestyle to support your child.

Read books, listen to podcasts, meet up with friends and family that will help to coach you. We all need coaching from people who have been there and moved through and experienced life's difficulties. Finding a life coach can be really helpful to work through some of these challenges. Look for someone to come alongside you who has compassion and understanding to show you empathy. You don't want them to pity you; you want to become empowered to take on this experience with self-assurance.

EXERCISE

Take the first step to getting fit and feeling good. Becoming fit parents really does help. It takes just twenty-one days to make a lifestyle change into a habit. And you can start with just ten minutes of exercise. That's right: in just ten minutes, you can reach an endorphin high that results in feeling happier, sleeping better, and thinking more clearly. Not only that, the endorphin boost can stay with you for two to three hours. If you've had an unfortunate night with your child, exercise can help you recover and be fresh for the day.

Choose a physical exercise that you enjoy. I found a local pool that had an early morning swim and got up before the children. It got me out of the house. I had swum before I had children, and it was enjoyable to go back to doing something I really liked. Matthew enjoyed running with the children and doing Tai Chi.

Find physical exercise and times that are practical. If you can get out of the house and into nature, you have that added health benefit. Studies show that being in nature reduces stress (cortisol, the stress hormone, decreases). Just walking through the trees for fifteen minutes can lower your heart rate, slow your breathing, and restore your mind. When you return home, you will have the potential to be more productive because you can think more clearly.

If you can't get outside, you could start your day by exercising first thing in the morning next to the bed, stretching and doing some strength exercises. You might find an app to follow. Or you could go to a quiet place in the house for yoga or Tai Chi.

If you find you just can't fit in a workout, then go for a walk with your child in the stroller. If they can walk, make the daily walk with your child an additional workout. Both you and your child will benefit from being in nature and fresh air.

WHAT ENERGIZES YOU?

While I found parenthood extremely fulfilling, I found myself setting aside activities I had enjoyed before the birth of my children in order to dedicate more of my time to them. Reconnecting with meaningful activities can be a powerful healing tool for parents who have begun to trade their identity as an individual for an identity solely focused on their child's disability. Think: What are the things that you did before you were a parent that made you feel good? What regenerated you? Did it involve quiet time or being active and with people? Taking a break to do something that you enjoy will again help to sustain you for the future.

So how would you use the leisure time afforded to you in an ideal world? What are you missing most about your past life? Write down the answers by making a list of things you have done in the past. Don't hold back. Don't entertain the thought that you don't have the time now. Don't entertain the thought that it is not practical. Begin by putting it on the list. You can hope and dream.

This list might include knitting, sewing, podcasts, reading, coffee with friends, exercise or a sports activity, puzzles, or games.

Go through the list and categorize it. What made you feel really good? What could you do without? What did you love that isn't practical right now? Put these things on the "Dream Big" list. These things take time away from the home and will require you to wait for them, and/or they will require more planning. Start small and stay consistent. Choose something you can pick up and put down like reading a book, doing a puzzle, or creating something.

Your personal journey toward healing begins with giving yourself permission to look after yourself—every day. We have found this to be a significant factor in the story of families and children who have made great progress.

In fact, it's imperative that you do this. It's not easy to find the time or create the habit, but taking it one little step at a time is all that is required. You will go through periods when there will be less time for you and other times when life is a little simpler, and you can and should take advantage of these times.

Begin to create a little "toolbox" for yourself. By taking the first step to look after yourself, you will be a better parent, better partner, better in your relationships, and certainly move toward restoring yourself.

DREAMS

We all have dreams, and with our dreams come disappointment when they don't happen the way we had hoped. As parents, we dream of what our family will be like, and this can often be a picture-book version. When reality hits, it just does not look that way. When things are even more out of the norm, there can be additional feelings of profound disappointment—deep and seemingly unrelenting sadness. This loss of our hopes and dreams leaves feelings of confusion and dread for the future.

Every parent has dreams for what their child's life will look like. Just as importantly, every parent imagines what the addition of a new child will mean for themselves and their family. When a child is slightly behind, injured, or born with a debilitating illness, those dreams seem so far from reality that parents often abandon them completely and can't seem to engage in the process of dreaming any longer.

Please don't stop dreaming.

Sometimes dreams need to change or be adjusted, but we must keep having them. You are allowed to dream and hope for your child. Dreams and goals are what keep us going. Both you and your child need them. We have over the years seen so many beautiful dreams come true in the families we have worked with. Children walking down the aisle as a bridesmaid in a wedding. They walked carefully and wore the most fashionable boots possible (not little ballet slippers), but they did it! Going on a hike with a team that carried them up the mountain but contributing in some way, and everyone enjoying every bit of being part of the experience and the team.

The dream you had as a parent for your child/children, because of the circumstances, can be reframed and will look different—this makes perfect sense.

I had hopes and dreams of taking my children on many day trips when they were younger, but this did not happen nearly as much as I had hoped as our days were filled with very important neurological stimulation. Now, though, much later, I see them experiencing life and having these adventures, and I appreciate these with deeper joy.

Dreams become recalibrated and they will happen in a different way. Maybe due to the challenges your child has, things need to be broken into steps, and consequently you will have mini dreams fulfilled rather than the big ones.

FAMILY SUCCESS STORY

If you were ever told that your child is incapable or have been force-fed a "doom and gloom" prognosis, then it is time to remove those professionals from your roster and sign on new talent!

We are a family of six. My husband and I have four children. Our second child, Ben, started receiving services for autism at age two and a half. We were very proactive and diligent in seeking therapies and advice from the best, but after nine years of speech, occupational, physical, and behavioral therapies, Ben, at age eleven and a half, still struggled immensely and was functioning at 35 percent brain function, or as a two- to three-year-old.

Our two biggest fears when considering traveling to the Family Hope Center were: *Is Ben too old? and Are we strong enough to even try?* Fear can be quite crippling and it's not easy to keep trying, but our family couldn't deny our feelings of discontent and restlessness.

I wanted to go to the movies or church without having an emergency exit plan. I wanted my son to have the internal motivation to do things for himself and others, and not constantly have to bribe him with screen time or treats. I wanted him to learn to ride a bike, tie his shoes, bathe himself, create stories, respect people's things, and engage with his family.

After nine years of conventional therapies, none of those goals were achieved. The unmanageable cost for these therapies and the lack of results were debilitating.

Ben's behaviors of erratic sleep, impulsiveness, self-injurious behaviors, and indifference to any discipline were creating resentment within our family. The countless meltdowns, the self-biting, the repetitive screeching, and our inability to do things as a family were all depleting our desire to try. We knew more was possible; we just had no idea how to achieve it.

But by the grace of God, we attended the Family Hope Center Parent Training Conference. By the third and final day of the conference, my husband and I had a renewed purpose. We started to learn how to be part of the solution, instead of part of the problem.

For the last five years we have been implementing the comprehensive neurological approach designed by the FHC team. We as a family have witnessed neuroplasticity and continue to see that growth is possible, no matter the age!

We as a family have the clarity of discernment and we are no longer fearful. We know our power. We know the brain grows when a family rallies behind the one struggling and stands united in implementing an evidence-based systematic approach in a loving home.

Ben is now sixteen years old and at the brain development of an eight- to nine-year-old. He is independently bathing, riding a bike, tying his shoes, writing and reading, balancing a checkbook, doing chores, running, playing sports, and so much more.

Ben has taught us about love, forgiveness, and service.

Allow your child to lead you. Be the change they need to thrive! Be strengthened and supported by the FHC team as you do the work and reap the rewards.

God bless you all.

—The Thompson Family

NEURO-PARENTING POINTS

- When looking after a child with special needs, parents become a distant second in terms of self-care and personal growth. This is normal, but it is also possible to create change and balance in your life.
- Be kind to yourself and remember—it's about your child's brain. You are the solution to your child's neurological challenges and can thrive within this challenge.
- Practice good nutrition habits. When busy and stressed, there's a tendency to gravitate to foods that make us feel good in the moment but nutritionally lack what the body and the brain need to function well.
- For optimum health and efficiency, the brain and body require seven to eight hours of sleep every night. Anything less can lead to sleep deprivation, which depletes your energy and focus. Find ways to get proper rest and a nap when you can.
- Celebrate small victories. Take time to acknowledge how far you have come, how much you have learned, and the great changes that you have made to your lifestyle to support your child and family.
- Get physical. Choose an exercise that you enjoy and find a practical time to do it daily. Even a ten-minute workout can provide

an endorphin boost that will result in feeling happier, sleeping better, and thinking clearer.

- Think about hobbies and activities that you once enjoyed and explore ways to pursue them again!
- New dreams and hopes can be reframed or happen in a new or different way, but they can still be realized.

CHAPTER 9

GROWING TOGETHER AS A FAMILY

We are writing this chapter not as professionals, but more as a dad and a mom who worked through this part of our lives and had the intention to keep moving forward—praying, trying, readjusting, growing, and executing the plan for our daughters' healing. We have seen many high-spirited families who figured out a healthy balance between their marriage and the family. What follows is the collective perspective on what we learned.

Whether your child with special needs is your only child, or your first, last, or mixed in the middle among other siblings, the extra time they require will strain you, the rest of the family, and all your relationships. So comes the challenge for the parents of finding a sense of balance within the family. Finding that balance can take a lifetime to achieve. You may feel like you are constantly juggling and asking the questions "Who needs me today?" or "Who needs me next?"

Of course, the objective is to grow into an integrated, thriving family, and find continuous ways to coach, guide, and support each family member to grow.

PARTNERSHIP

This is the primary relationship and should not be put to the side. You and your partner can become stronger together as you become a united team raising your family together. This relationship needs attention for multiple reasons. First, this relationship is the foundation on which you build your family. Second, you will be setting an example for your children on how to work on relationships by demonstrating your love and support for each other.

It is way too easy to find a child's needs consume all our time in the week. This can take over all your partner time together. There may be a temptation to separate and divide tasks and roles both in and out of the home. While this may be necessary, when you can do things together or share in elements of the home and childcare and therapy, it strengthens your relationship. Simultaneously, the child benefits from being able to work with and relate to each of you.

Finding time to sit and talk is certainly a challenge, but scheduling it to happen at least once each week is a beginning. If you don't put it on the schedule at least once a week and block out the time, it probably won't happen. Tell the children that Mommy and Daddy have a meeting now and they are not to be interrupted. They will most likely try to gain your attention, and you will need to take some time for them to learn to wait their turn.

Listen to each other, and take turns relating how your week has been. You might find you are too tired to be spontaneous, so prepare an agenda of what you want to ask each other. Discuss how time is going for each of you overall.

Just the awareness of being heard and supported can often be enough to move forward and not get stuck emotionally. The more you do this, the more you get to know each other, know how your partner is doing, what it is you are each struggling with, and how to support each other.

By meeting to talk with regularity, you are more likely to keep ahead of any challenges. If issues arise, be sure you build in extra time to address these concerns and problems, and work through them—don't try to cram it all into one meeting. Give it the time it needs.

Once you connect on a personal level—so important but overlooked—you can move on to talking about the children and how the week went. Become united together in the direction for each child and the family as a whole, and set new goals and review the progress toward the existing goals. You can do this.

What isn't practical today can certainly be put down as a goal for the future. Going on a date may seem way out of reach now, but planning for a date can often be just as fun as the date itself. While going out on a date is nice, we found taking the time for each other and being creative in the home was more doable. These became fun experiences we look back at fondly. The advantages: They didn't require money for a babysitter or a show or restaurant. Just some planning. We would put the children to bed early and let them know this was our special time together. However, they often broke those rules, and we would try not to let them see us smiling as they would sneak out of bed to get a peek at the table set with candles and us holding hands and chatting together without them.

When we could, going out was also put on the schedule. Children seeing their parents dressed up and going out for a good time is a great example of how a relationship grows.

FAMILY INVOLVEMENT: SIBLINGS

Some of the questions we frequently hear from parents: "What about the siblings?" "How will they feel about the time we spend with their sister?" "Won't they be jealous?" "Won't they be angry?" and "Will they feel neglected?"

Parents often carry added guilt related to feeling the need to balance the time spent with each child. As they witness your devotion to their sibling, your children learn that in this family they will be given the help needed when they need it and develop a full sense of security.

SADNESS FOR ALL THE FAMILY

For legitimate reasons, parents often want to protect siblings from what is happening. Unfortunately, in reality, this isn't possible. They feel sad just like you: they feel your grief, and their own sense of grief. They also feel fear and concern, no matter the age of the child. In fact, even babies can and will feel sadness.

Older siblings have expressed their frustration and sadness over their unsuccessful efforts to try to play or engage with their siblings. They have even expressed their embarrassment of their sibling's behavior, particularly when out of the home together. These are real concerns and challenges. So what do you do to avoid a sibling remaining sad, feeling separated, angry, and even anxious?

You include them.

Keeping everyone informed about the basics can lead to overall understanding. Explain what's happening, the problems and challenges, and the solutions at that time. Keep it simple. Remember the age of the child. The details aren't usually needed with younger children. Take away the mystery surrounding their sibling with special needs by giving factual explanations about the brain and how you are working to grow and develop the brain. Also, of course, breathe and take the time to listen, encouraging questions and asking them what they want to know and what they might be concerned about. Your other children will learn that rocky times and sadness come and go through life, but we can get through those times and end up more emotionally resilient as individuals and as a strong, united family.

WAYS TO BE ORGANIZED AND CREATE ROUTINES AND EXPECTATIONS FOR ALL

While the focus is on helping the child with special needs, including the siblings in the healing process over time helps them develop empathy.

It might slow you down as they learn to assist and participate, but the benefits far outweigh the time it takes to guide and instruct your well child.

Any guilt you might be feeling that the siblings are getting lost in the shuffle will be replaced with the confidence of knowing you are empowering them, and that they are now part of the care and therapy.

To be sure this goes well, it will require some organization on your part. Structure the environment to include each child. They should know what is expected of them, how to complete their role, and when they need to be present. This will give each child a secure and stable base.

We would also recommend setting clear goals and objectives for the tasks and responsibilities they have. Structure the layout of the day for yourself and each family member. Writing it as a list that includes everyone in the family, including parents, or in book form, or in a posted chart, are some options. Be careful about getting ahead of yourself. Often, things can look great on paper but are too complicated to execute. Only do what you feel will be helpful and begin with one thing at a time for each family member.

When preparing for what tasks to give to each child, consider:

- Their age—no matter the age, they can be involved.
  - They could get materials or hold materials between the stimulation exercises.

- What is their skill level, and where would they be best helping you?
  - Some children who can work independently might be best to handle household chores so you can keep working with your child. Be sure they first connect with you and their sibling with a hug and kiss before they go off to their important role.

- Is the role purposeful? If it is not, they will see through it and not feel validated.
- Assign the task with clarity.
- Practice and coach them until they master the task.
- If quality drops a little, and it will, step back in. The benefits of involvement are key to learning.

The way you organize and introduce this depends on the age of each child. It is helpful and vital for them to feel like they are part of the solution. Over time, they will gradually begin to realize how important they are to their sibling's success—even gaining improved self-worth from contributing to their sibling's development.

WAYS TO STAY POSITIVE AND ENCOURAGED

We all need encouragement. You and the family will benefit from finding ways to celebrate and acknowledge success and progress, however small. It's easy to be caught up in the business of the day and miss seeing the changes, or have those changes become the norm, and thereby harder to observe.

Proactively looking for ways to encourage all the family to participate and contribute can feel like an added burden. Breathe and take a step back. Focus on finding ways to respond with positivity. Look for ways to find the positive in the little moments of the day and acknowledge them out loud. For some of you, this will be hard work, but as you focus on it more, a good and important habit will develop. It will help your partner, your children, and you.

Cultivate ways to celebrate milestones. Not just the big ones but all the little ways you see change. If your child had one less tantrum or one less seizure this week, we can be tempted to think or even say, "My child still has tantrums," or we can celebrate it and say, "My child had one less tantrum this week."

When a child's behavior is a challenge, we can feel like we are always correcting. Take on the challenge of "I caught you doing something good." You will need to be one step ahead of the child to be able to jump in with a positive comment before they have the time to do or say something negative.

Tracking the positive changes in a form that's manageable helps everyone in the family. A victory board is ideal, as it's always there for everyone to see. All changes, however small, should be placed on the board.

Documenting all new abilities is very important. Remember that many small positives outweigh one big negative, so recording victories for the child with special needs, as well as each family member, becomes a great encouragement. You can record anything.

Hand out cards that say "I caught you doing something good," or smiley-face tokens.

Keep a notebook close by or track it on your phone. If you focus on every time your child is sick, you might miss the fact that they are improving in their overall health. Start documenting every day they are healthy. Then maybe the days of sickness won't seem so bad.

You can turn any negative into a positive. For every negative thing that happens to us, we need five positives to replace it. So if you can stay ahead of the curve, it will help you resist getting knocked down by the negatives when they come.

BEHAVIORS AND RULES OF ENGAGEMENT

When two adults join together and start a family, they each bring a unique set of life experiences into the newly developing family. This includes traditions that become adopted into the new family; some become merged, but you also may develop unique ones. Along with the family traditions, each partner comes with a package of standards and values that were modeled for them. Some of those are important to you and, if they are not followed by your partner, can become a source of irritation. Others, you may want to change for various reasons. It is important to take time early on in your relationship to share these values with each other. Like the traditions, establishing a joint effort of what is and is not important to each of you becomes a very important point.

Have you established the "Rules of Engagement" within your family?

Traditions create enjoyment and memories for us. Rules create security for all of your children and are an important point for their development. When children do not have clear boundaries, they will be more inclined to test you until they feel you have drawn the line for them. They need to know what you expect of them. Without a clear reference point, they can feel and behave in a disorganized fashion. For the child with special needs, this will be amplified.

So step one is to take the time to discuss each of your differences. What is important to each of you? Most likely, one of you tends to be more relaxed and the other may tend to be more rigid. Clear boundaries are there for safety and security, just like road signs and traffic lights. For the sake of the children, you both need to decide the way you want to set the rules. Children desperately need this consistency, or they will not know the boundaries.

We have seen many families face a behavioral challenge with very different strategies on how to solve it and what the consequences should be for the child. They agree to follow one parent's ideas first for a period of time. Then, if that doesn't work, they try the other way. Try not to take it personally if your strategy does not work but your partner's does, as this approach often leads to overall success because both parents are united and respect each other's view. Outside support can often be necessary to address challenging behaviors, and we would absolutely recommend this. In our family, we referenced other ideas constantly to make sure we were thinking clearly.

With these basics in place, let's talk about the child with special needs. Do you have the same expectations with this child as you do with the other children in the family? We often find that the standards are different. This can be because the parents are unsure that the child can handle boundaries due to lack of ability. Unfortunately, this can lead to sympathy rather than support. Your goal is to include the child with special needs within the family. They need clearly set boundaries to follow, and those boundaries and expectations should be the same as the other children, so begin with the same expectations. Follow through and teach the boundaries in the moment. Be extra clear, take your time, and recognize that your child with special needs will need way more time and frequency than the typical child before they learn. But by consistently teaching in the moment, your child with special needs will begin to understand the point and learn.

Use your child developmental chart (IDPC) to guide you in the implementation. You want to look at two key factors: their age in their understanding and their age in emotional development. Look at the difference between the neurological age and the chronological age in these two functions. What is the discrepancy between the two? This reality check can help you to know if your expectations—or the way you are trying to implement and teach these boundaries—are in line with your child's capabilities. If you have a ten-year-old with the emotional age of a two-year-old, they can't be expected to do things independently. Two-year-olds always need a parent close by to keep them safe, guide them, teach them, and prevent them from doing things that are dangerous. As a parent, learning to stay close and guide in a supportive way without too many words is a valuable skill that can't be overemphasized. Just try it. Go to your child and give them instructions. Stay there directing them with a point or a hand on the shoulder. Wait, go with them, and stay close as they complete the task. Speak only after the instruction or task is completed. This is quite effective, more often than not.

Remember, too, that consequences are needed for children to learn that they have crossed a boundary. Again, you should be thinking of the child's neurological age when choosing effective and understood consequences.

We hear many comments and concerns from parents who don't know what the best consequences might be for a particular challenge. They feel as if they have tried everything. They wonder about time-outs and other specific consequences. They just do not comprehend how one simple correction with a neurotypical sibling can be quickly turned into the child learning and changing, while the child with special needs has not changed after multiple repetitions.

First, consider whether you're using a consequence appropriate to the neurological age of the child. For example, if you are using a time-out (or pausing for thinking time) that is too long, by the time it is over, your child may have forgotten what the time-out was for. As a neurological principle, your child needs frequency to learn from the consequences.

You might need to repeat a short time-out multiple times for your child to even begin to learn.

Time-outs vary. For example, if your child is throwing food, you can opt to remove the food rather than removing the child from the table. You might hold their hands to prevent them from throwing the food. When the child struggles with picturing/thinking about something they did, they learn better right in the moment rather than having to think about it in a separate room. Children with special needs often do not have the ability to keep in mind what is/was happening in another room.

Keep your instructions simple. Just state that you understand them but do not get too wordy. They will learn best with actions rather than words.

Enlist the siblings by explaining your goals and their roles. They will feel empowered as they have a clear purpose in the process toward the family goal. The siblings do not need to understand all the differences and details. But explaining that their sister requires a different path for learning is helpful. They can be encouraged to be helpful by demonstrating behavior that can be modeled.

A good example of this would be eating separately. As discussed in the previous chapter, you need to be able to eat with an element of peace, and this also applies to the rest of the family. Your family goal, ultimately, is to have a family meal. If this is not yet possible, here are some suggestions and ways to break this down into steps and small goals.

- One parent focuses on the child.
- The child can sit at the table as long as he is not disruptive.
- The child eats before the rest of the family eats, if this makes the most sense.
- The child joins the meal for a few minutes at the beginning or end of the meal while the family eats, with full parental support.
- During the meal, the child can be alone if safe or with one parent.
- The siblings set examples through the meal of how to use utensils, sit nicely, have a conversation, etc.

HANDLING CONFLICT

If your child with special needs has challenging behavior, the priority is always safety—for themselves, siblings, and others. If anyone does not feel both physical and emotional safety, then adjustments must quickly be implemented. Avoid times when your children are left unattended. You may need to keep them separate when you cannot be present.

You as the parent need to take the lead here. Don't expect the other children to take on this responsibility. In fact, you should make it clear that it is your role and that they cannot take over your role. Encourage them to lead by example and come and get you when they need you. Be specific as to when they should summon you. If things are not working out, then stay close at hand so you can keep watch and step in to coach in the moment. Young children and neurologically young children will forget quickly, so discussing after the event is too late for them. They need to learn immediately.

There will be conflict along the way—it's all part of a growing family. Conflict is normal, so when it does happen, take a step back and work toward teaching and resolving it with understanding and sensitivity. Understand the age of the child/children who are part of the conflict. You will be able to address this challenge with a firm and clear approach that includes the compassion you have for the children involved.

FAMILY TIME—DOING THINGS TOGETHER

Family vacations, playing games, participating in sports, going to museums—these are all things you may have done in your family growing up. Or maybe they're things you feel you missed out on and you now want to experience with your family. As we talked about in the previous chapter, these hopes and dreams can still be on your list, but finding ways to adjust to the current circumstances within a family with a child with special needs becomes very important.

IN THE HOME

Having a specific playtime each day can be helpful when the child with special needs does not play and interact well. Parents, siblings, and the child with special needs will all need to learn successful interactive play. One thing we do know is that the brothers and sisters have the desire to play with their sibling, and they are sad that they cannot figure it out.

We all need to learn that what comes naturally for the siblings and others does not come naturally for this child. It can, however, be taught by you and learned by the child—remember, it takes frequency, intensity, and duration matching the intellectual and emotional age of the child. Start small with a specific game. One that really seems to work well is rolling a ball back and forth. The child with special needs will need one parent to be behind them, and the sibling must know how close to be, when to roll the ball back, and how much she must slow down. Your role as the parent is to be sure they are close enough to each other for success and engagement; keep the game going with some hand-over-hand support if need be. Keeping each child in the game can be a challenge, and you may need to bring them back. Try for five minutes (it can feel like an eternity). You may find that this is the longest game you ever played together. You may find that the engagement comes and goes, and this is typical.

Set aside time each day to be with each child in the family. It may be a conversation or an activity or help with homework. This time needs to be scheduled and planned. It needs to become uninterrupted time. The child who gets the attention needs to really feel that it's their time. If you keep your attention on them when interruptions come—like a ringing cell phone or another child interrupting—they feel special. This will also teach the other child not to interrupt. As parents divide and delegate to each other, you can eventually facilitate this time in the family. This may be an occasion for one parent to stay separately with the child with special needs.

Whether big or small, working out ways and schedules to have special family time together is crucial for the overall mental health of each family member and of the family as a whole.

OUTSIDE THE HOME

For good reason, we see many of our families avoiding going out with their child with special needs. If you are one of those families and your child has unwanted behavior or tantrums when out, or you want to protect them from germs due to their weakened immune system, or you're afraid they will run away, you have good reason to pause before going out in public. Some children might be okay when out, but when they return home, the overstimulation results in hyperactivity or having a meltdown. It's important to know that even if going out now seems like an impossibility, it's a doable activity for the future with some structure and neurological organization.

Many of our parents struggle with managing the day-to-day errands that need to happen outside the home in order for the home to function. Including the children in these activities provides excellent learning and bonding time for a neurotypical child, but that's not always the case with a child with special needs. While going through this phase, take a "divide and conquer" approach until the child is ready neurologically to gain a benefit from joining you.

As an example, shopping can really be problematic. Here are some strategies we've seen our parents take to ease that stress:

- One parent goes out shopping while the other stays home.
- Sometimes the child with special needs does well when shopping with Dad as he has not seen him all week, so this becomes a Dad/child activity.
- Shop for only one hour (or less) at one store.
- Create a homemade book of the store you are going to and include the behavior that you want all the children to follow. Carry the book with you and review frequently if needed.

Overall, when planning to introduce an outside activity that includes the child with special needs, it's important to begin with small activities. Rehearse at home, making it as real as possible, and with plenty of frequency, until you feel it is time for a trial run. When you do go out, assign one parent to give full support and guidance to the child. This parent might need to be ready to take the child for short breaks or return home before the others.

Whether it's an activity at home or outside the home, do the same activity regularly enough for the child to master before adding in a variation. When the siblings are part of the activity, they should be included in the preparation and practice and know their roles. Are they modeling or being an example? Do they need to slow down or wait for their sister or brother?

FAMILY TIME SEPARATELY

When including the child with special needs in family activities isn't yet possible, it's important to have family time together with the rest of the family. At first, parents may feel sad and guilty leaving the child at home, and struggle with feeling the need to include everyone. We have seen that there are many benefits to separating.

Your child with special needs requires a routine. When you go out, the routine is changed, and this can be disruptive. When the child is left home and kept on their routine, they are actually much happier for it. This, in turn, makes the family happier.

The other children benefit from the attention they receive when one or both parents are not focused on the child who needs constant attention as well. This is their opportunity to build their relationship with their parents. It's also a time when they can move through an activity or experience at a pace that works for them, as they don't need to slow down for their sibling.

We have seen so many families over the years and watched as their children grew. Some families chose each year to take family vacations with the siblings left at home. Others resisted this for several years. We have been privileged to watch these families grow together and become strong and united teams who love and support each other.

We remember one family who really wanted to take a trip to Italy, as their girls were ready for that adventure. They made the decision to leave the younger, special-needs daughter home as it was just going to be too much for her. Not only did the parents and their girls have a wonderful trip doing things together, they also returned home to a very happy daughter who had been at home following her routine.

FAMILY SUCCESS STORY

Our family dynamic really plays an integral part in our daughter Bailey's therapy program. With four children, schedules in our house, like most, can be very busy. We, as parents of a hurt child, understand how easy it is for the well siblings to feel devalued when working one-on-one so much with their hurt sister. We elected to let them be a team player versus a spectator in her development, and it has proven to be a hugely valuable application for our entire family of six!

Even at the young age of six, our Abigail participates in sign language, entertainment while Bailey is in the orthopedic stander, and even likes to coordinate her baby dolls down the inclined floor (correctly!). Our eldest two daughters, who are ten and twelve, are just as helpful as adults would be. The one-on-one time the girls have with Bailey allows for wonderful bonding time, not to mention awesome backups when Mom or Dad are really in need of a quick assistant!

Burnout can still happen to us, even in this dynamic, though we try our best to prevent it. We find taking a day off once a week, or even a day when we just need to organize other parts of our lives, allows us to have a much clearer focus for the days ahead.

Lastly, it is most important for Mom and Dad to be a team. When something isn't working, like many things in a relationship, communication is our key to resolving it.

—*The Czar Family*

NEURO-PARENTING POINTS

- Parents, as partners, succeed when focusing on being stronger and united in raising a family together. This relationship is the foundation on which you build your family and help your child, and it sets a positive example to your children about love and support.
- The child with special needs naturally consumes additional time and energy, so this must be kept in balance with time as a couple and with other children in the household.
- It is a very positive action to plan to make time—at least once a week—to discuss family matters and personal needs and goals, individually and as a couple.
- When there are other children at home, planning quality time, both one-on-one and together, is very wise. It is also valuable to explain the challenges of the child with special needs in a way that is age appropriate, so the siblings understand what is happening and why, and how they can be of help and support.
- Endeavor to lead by example so that every child in the family can grow, exhibit patience and compassion, and learn how to solve problems.
- Establish tasks and routines for each child and allow the children to participate in the brain-based exercises and activities you do with the child with special needs.
- Focusing on and keeping track of small accomplishments and victories while celebrating milestones will help maintain a positive attitude.
- When problems or challenges arise, be firm, clear, and consistent. Turn every challenge into a teachable moment.
- Set a specific time each day to engage with all the children and do something fun together.
- Plan time together with the children separately. Many children with special needs are more comfortable in their home environment and are happier staying home with a caregiver.

CHAPTER 10

BUILDING A SUPPORT TEAM

Alone we can do so little; together we can do so much.

—Helen Keller

I n chapters eight and nine we emphasized taking care of yourself and strengthening your family relationships. After these core elements are established and
flowing fairly well—or as well as can be—the other long-term, critical element is building your support team. Being able to rely on a unified team that
cooperatively supports you and your child's efforts toward growth and development is crucial. We want to share a collection of ideas and concepts we've seen
successfully implemented over the years—all in hopes of helping your family
gain another level of support and strength.

Anyone that respects your goals or knows you and loves your child can form
the basis of your team, which might include doctors, therapists, teachers, grandparents, babysitters, close friends, and anyone else who may already be playing

an active role in your child's care and support. As our medical director, Dr. Kristin Clague Reihman, always says, "As it turns out, life is a team sport."

WHAT TO CONSIDER BEFORE BUILDING YOUR TEAM

Your support team doesn't have to be large. When you think of a team, you probably think of three to six members. Team size is contingent on your situation and your child's unique needs. You can choose as many or as few people as you feel are necessary. And you can increase and decrease your team's size based on what's happening in your family and your child's life anytime.

Consider each candidate and choose wisely and conscientiously. Team members should be positive and cheerful people who are reliable and demonstrate attention to detail. Whether you've interviewed an outside candidate or talked at length with someone familiar or close to you, confirm they understand and support your hopes and goals for your child. Most of all, they should believe, like you, that it's possible for your child to make improvement and heal.

On the professional side, you may want to include physical and occupational therapists, teachers, and perhaps your child's pediatrician or specialist. While many of these people won't meet daily with your child, their alignment with your goals is invaluable to your child's overall well-being.

After a few months have passed, examine how the team is getting along and supporting you to be effective and efficient in assisting your child and in helping you balance your time wisely within your family. Team members who listen, follow your lead, offer wise suggestions, and proactively fill holes you didn't anticipate are golden. If you feel someone isn't quite working out in the role you've agreed on, don't feel awkward about adjusting or replacing them. Just politely and generously thank them for their time and assistance. As long as each member of your team continues to understand their role and support the big picture, you'll reap the rewards of their service by watching your child develop.

Having an excellent team in place will help you make sustainable progress with your child's development. You will be in a better position to make decisions, obtain answers, and get help when you need it. Lastly, you will feel less alone and exhausted, which is invaluable.

WHERE TO FIND THE HELP YOU NEED

The first place you'll want to look is toward your immediate family. That might include your other children if they're mature enough. In our experience, we've found grandparents, if available, will be particularly helpful and willing to be part of the team, too. You might also consider reaching out to extended family members who live nearby. These can include sisters and brothers, aunts and uncles, nieces and nephews. Try not to be too timid to ask for their assistance. Many members of your family may actually want to help but feel unsure about asking you.

When you speak with your family, be clear about what you need. Explain, in exact terms, what you will request from them and let them know it's okay to say no if they don't feel up to the task. This isn't a situation where anyone should take part out of guilt or obligation. Some family members, even though they know and care about you and your child, might not be able to help at this time, though they may be able to assist you in some way in the future. It's far better to excuse them than apply pressure and force them into saying yes, which can lead to regrets and resentment later.

Look to your close friends next. Provided they have the time, close friends generally have your (and your child's) interests at heart. In fact, many may have already demonstrated their support to you in other ways. Again, make sure to explain what you need and the roles you need fulfilled so they understand how they fit in the picture.

After close family and friends, consider approaching a few professionals you know well and trust. These can include doctors, teachers and teacher's aides, physical and occupational therapists, or special-needs caretakers. Many of these great professionals may have limited time to help out, but if they express interest, explore ways to make it work even if they are only available to consult with you periodically.

Let's say you find family, friends, and professionals aren't in a position to join your team due to problems with logistics, schedules, or other personal and professional obligations. It happens. Don't be discouraged. There are other resources to consider when building a team. Our advice:

- Seek recommendations from family and friends. Trusted family members and friends can be a well of connections and resources—don't be shy about tapping into their contacts.

- Network at your religious institution. Even if you don't regularly attend religious services or functions, these spiritual communities can be immensely supportive and helpful. Please don't hesitate to reach out and seek help from these congregations.

- Tap into community centers, clubs, and social acquaintances. Do you frequent your local YMCA or YWCA, JCC, Kiwanis club, or country club? Do you belong to a book club or a gym? Think of acquaintances you have whom you can approach or network with who might help or offer referrals.

- Enlist high school and college students. Contact local high schools, colleges, and community colleges to see if there are students who may be interested in participating. Many high school juniors or seniors are required to do community work or senior projects; college students may be studying to become physical education teachers, healthcare practitioners, special education teachers, PTs, or OTs, and would find the experience valuable to their education and training. Some students might even be able to attain degree credits in the process.

- Check with public safety service retirees. Do not overlook retired schoolteachers, officers, and former firefighters and first responders. In our experience, many of these individuals are eager and receptive to volunteering their time, and they offer an added benefit—experience in problem-solving, or certification in CPR and other health, safety, or emergency training that can

be of value and relief to you, especially if your child has compromised health, limited abilities, or is prone to seizures.

At the end of the day, don't be afraid to reach out and ask—there are
more people out there to support you than you think!

CHOOSING YOUR TEAM AND MANAGING EXPECTATIONS

Make sure that everyone has a role for which they are suited and able.
Find out what people's skills are, what they like to do, and then ask
them how they would like to contribute. Once you have this conversation, you can decide how to integrate them and what you want them to
accomplish.

Will they be good caregivers? If so, their role can be to watch, play
with, or read to your child or watch your other kids. Are they organized
and flexible? If so, they can run errands, pick up your kids from school or
practice when you are stuck for time, go grocery shopping, or even help
clean your house. Over the years, we've been amazed at the wonderful stories of team members selflessly doing the big things and the little things to
help and support families.

Sit down with your partner and carefully map out each team member's
time wisely, including your own. Try to create a balanced routine so that
your "A-team" can fully support you and your child, help supplement your
responsibilities, and give you some time to breathe. Each member of your
team should have a particular role and a purpose and should know what
that role is. You or your team leader will coordinate what each person does
and when. Define what and whom you need and find the right hero to fill
the role. The adage that "less is more" can sometimes apply here. Begin
with a small, manageable team with clear expectations and scale up when
needed.

Once your team members get used to how they can effectively help you
and your child, it's essential to routinely keep them informed. This can be

hard when balancing so many hectic schedules. Using a WhatsApp group text to communicate, send photos, leave messages, and give a shout-out with today's victory is perfect for team cohesion and spirit.

Many of our families show their gratitude and appreciation by hosting a barbecue, having a Christmas get-together, or some other event where their team members can come together, get to know each other, talk about their specific roles, and have some fun.

MAKING CHANGES TO YOUR TEAM

Even if you feel you have the best team in place, situations may change, or outside influences may occur that can make it necessary to reduce the number of team members. Regardless of the circumstances, which can sometimes be awkward, change may be necessary and productive. If you have a strong team leader, make the change together. If your instincts tell you that something doesn't feel right, then gently make the change. Your energy will be better spent moving forward rather than adapting and managing the team member that needs to be released.

Every family we have worked with experiences these moments. The best families make the change quickly when they deem it necessary.

Once you have your team in place, give it a few months before you reassess. As in most jobs, three months is a typical adjustment period to see how things are working. This goes both ways, of course. You'll have a chance to evaluate who's a good fit (or not), and each member can also decide if staying on the team is right for them as well.

If your child's stage of development has changed, you might also need to make an adjustment to the team or to each person's responsibilities. You may have to expand or contract your team. Again, this is common.

Whether your team members are volunteers or paid, conducting a quarterly assessment is valuable. If you let too much time pass, it becomes more difficult to make the changes you need. Let every-one on your team know that you plan to evaluate the team every three months. This way, if things are not optimal, you can part ways on mutually agreeable terms with no hard feelings.

WORKING WITH PROFESSIONALS

Professionals who work with or help your child can be part of your support team. Even if they are not a part of your daily/weekly routine, you still want to ensure that you have the right people on your side. Geography, financial resources, and health insurance restrictions can limit your access to or scope of appropriate care. While you can't always handpick your child's teacher or specialist, you can work to build respectful relationships with those who care for your child.

QUESTIONS TO ASK WHEN CHOOSING MEDICAL PROFESSIONALS

When interviewing and choosing professionals, ask how they plan to help your child. Find out about their approach to wellness. The most important consideration is whether their principles of healing are in alignment with your principles and approach.

Are they committed to:

- Healing the root cause of your child's condition?
- Natural healing at all times, rather than defaulting to antibiotics and medications?
- Taking a physiology approach rather than a pathology approach to healing?
- Parental involvement and consideration in every discussion?

Be mindful of the expertise of each professional and be careful not to have false expectations. Strive to keep your questions targeted to the expertise of that professional. Ask and then listen. If he or she is open-minded and accommodating, great! If not, it's best to move on. With time and effort, we are confident you will eventually find another professional who fits.

Always remember that you're in the driver's seat. You're interviewing them, not the other way around. You need professionals who are 100 percent dedicated to healing.

PARENT SUPPORT GROUPS

Support groups geared to special-needs parents can be a great source of comfort and information. They provide a safe and potentially informed environment in which to share experiences and ideas, discuss common challenges and solutions, and exchange resources like doctors, therapists, classes, and services. For parents who feel alone, isolated, or lacking the camaraderie of like-minded people, joining a group can be very comforting. In fact, many groups go beyond their regularly scheduled meetings and have family days, outings, barbecues, and social events. They can also be a place where strong and lasting friendships are cultivated.

Most towns have support groups for special-needs parents. You can find them through the professionals with whom you're working, as well as through your church, library, community center, or online. You can also find groups through organizations that support and advocate for children with specific diagnoses, whether autism spectrum disorders, cerebral palsy, or ADD/ADHD.

For those residing outside major cities, take heart—online communities of special-needs parents are abundant and thriving. A simple search will connect you with other parents across your town, state, region, or country. Many of these groups can be found on social media platforms like Facebook. You can check out these groups and see which are the most suitable.

It's best to align yourself with other parents and groups who are positive, proactive, and physiologically centered. Ideally, you want to be among people with whom you can share ideas and feel invigorated by. Once you're in a group for several months, assess how well the group is serving you. Are the members open-minded? Will they support what you're doing for your child? Are they in the same place as you philosophically? If, at any time, you begin to harbor doubts, consider moving on to another group.

SCHOOLS AND LEARNING ENVIRONMENTS

What type of school or support system would most benefit your child? This is a big question filled with challenges and uncertainties. The answer depends on several factors, including:

- Knowing your child's neurological age (through the IDPC chart results)
- Your child's aptitude for learning
- Your child's comfort level being away from home and in a school environment
- Your child's ability to sit and focus for four or more hours a day
- The type of support and accommodation the school can provide that is both safe and individualized for your child's needs

To make an initial assessment—or to assess a child who is already attending school—you may also consider the following:

- Is school the right place for your child?
- Will your child do well in a classroom setting?
- Is your child comfortable in groups?
- Does your child have many needs that the school is not designed for or not equipped to meet?
- Is there a possibility that your child may get bullied?
- Does your child have the potential to make friends at school?
- Is your child or could your child get anxious about not keeping up?
- Is your child in school struggling to keep up academically?

If your child is already in school, does the school collaborate with you and support your child and your team? Be proactive. Go to the school and discuss ways you can collaborate. Tell them: "I want to work with you. I want to help you understand and better help my child. I want to better communicate with you about things."

If the school is unwilling to work with you, ultimately, it's not the ideal environment because you won't feel supported and run the risk that your needs will be undermined.

Positive collaboration is vital. If you're arguing more than succeeding, reconsider. Try your best not to denigrate the school system—it is not always equipped to work the way you need. Don't try to change the system or the school or insist that everything be done your way—this will almost always be met with resistance. Find another school or consider homeschooling.

When you are shopping for a proactive school or learning environment, ask if the school will allow you to sit in for a day to observe, and if it is possible to schedule time periodically to see your child in action. Collaborating and sharing ideas on behavior and learning will be extremely helpful for your child and the teacher. Most teachers want to know how you are successful with your child at home so they can duplicate these positive efforts.

Also, check to see if the school is open to adapting the day to suit your child. Could they come in late, leave early, or attend fewer days? If entering a new school, your child should be permitted to make a gradual transition into the classroom and the daily routine. Obviously, this is a complicated situation since your child's neurology and the new school's expertise may or may not be a great fit.

Look elsewhere if a school isn't working for your child. There may be specialized schools or programs that will be more appropriate for your child. If you can't find the right school or find that getting to a promising school creates a logistical nightmare, you might consider—as many of our parents do for a few years—homeschooling. While homeschooling may seem like a daunting alternative, every year, more and more special-needs parents find it to be the best option. We have coached thousands of parents into successfully creating a positive homeschooling environment and watched as they improved their child's neurological development. Like support groups, there are local, regional, and online communities that will provide the resources, tools, and connections you need to facilitate a homeschooling program. Home may turn out to be the most suitable, safe, productive, and viable environment for learning.

OTHER SUPPORT PEOPLE

Beyond your team, there may be others with particular knowledge, skills, or expertise you need to rely on. For example, you might consider hiring an advocate. This person is like a personal administrative assistant who can look after more complex, time-consuming issues that are of benefit for children with special needs. All states offer financial support to children who are classified with disabilities, and your advocate can check out what is available and help with whatever paperwork and filing is necessary to ensure that your child qualifies for and receives benefits. The same goes for dealing with Medicaid or helping you schedule an Individualized Education Program (IEP) assessment for your child at school.

A family lawyer can help you with setting up a trust, wills, estate planning, guardianships, and have your back if you run into problems with health insurance, discrimination, and other legal matters. Similarly, an accountant may also advise on ways to maximize your income taxes and your budget, and to maintain your cash flow.

We hope this information has been helpful. As always, you can also find support and resources through our Family Hope Center Facebook group, which is an ongoing resource for our families. We have many families worldwide who have found ways to successfully utilize their local community resources.

FAMILY SUCCESS STORY

We were given a gift. We didn't know what kind of gift this would end up being. It was definitely not what we expected for our fourth child. This particular little gift seemed bigger and more daunting than anything we had ever encountered in our family's history. This gift wasn't wrapped with clean, crisp, colorful wrapping paper and a nice curly ribbon. Victoria Joy came more like a tiny little envelope with a coupon that seemed to promise a difficult, unknown trip into the years to come. I can safely say that one of the reasons we could enjoy this gift the way we do is because we were given a lifeline.

Our lifeline was found at the end of a call to "the wrong number." I landed on the Family Hope Center's answering machine. An incessant and intense curiosity (in retrospect, a God-sent strong guiding emotion) to find out what organization it was made me call again and pursue them. We found out it was a place that could help people with "brain injuries." We asked a hundred questions and almost miraculously a couple of weeks later my husband and I walked into the three-day parent training seminar.

As a human, as a mom, and as a special ed teacher, my brain was exploding with new information. Do you mean we can grow the brain, that you know how to do it, and that you know how to get to it? You are going to teach us and mentor us through it, too?

We came home infused with hope and a new resolve to save our child and to change the world.

We had been beaten down with the realization of having a child "like this" mixed with all the practicality of appointments and abrupt schedule changes. Seizures every five minutes. Dispensing the medicine to stop the seizures. Trying to feed the eight-pound, eight-month-old child who sleeps too long because of the seizure medicine. Pumping breast milk. Feeding the milk through a feeding tube in the baby's nose that comes out when the baby throws up, and then trying to decide to give more medicine because she might have thrown it up. All of this sloppily stirred with the words of well-meaning doctors, who said, "This is pretty much what you're gonna have," sprinkled heavily with therapist visits. Meanwhile, deadlines for the other children's school and activities were falling through the cracks, and a marriage and home were needing nurturing, too.

Coming home every six months with a designed program for our child looked like a huge undertaking, but we had an official, comprehensive, "let's get out of this mess" plan, and we were going somewhere!

Having a program designed carefully for our daughter was and is such a gift. Sitting in a non-medical-looking office with professionals that asked questions like, "Is there anything else you want to tell me about your daughter?" was such a new idea for us who had been at countless appointments, where our daughter's name was on a chart with numbers and diagnosis but who was barely really the focus of things. Who asks questions like that? How come we are not rushing through an appointment? What a blessing!

We were given a program that would take hours to accomplish. What else were we to do? Let her just sit there in her chair looking cute but nothing else? We had a chance to help our child. Our daughter was blind, couldn't hear, and couldn't feel. We were all game. We sat the kids down and had a mini-neurology seminar and went to town. For Tori to learn how to hear, we had to tell the boys to "scare the baby like this" with pots and pans. For Tori to see, we had to make Tori's pupils dilate and constrict and shine the light in her eyes "like this." For Tori to feel, we had to brush her little body "like this."

We had plenty of seasons that worked and some that didn't. Times we had to rally the community to come help (three faithful volunteers coming through our doors two times a day), and times when the home was too busy and needed a stretch where we did all the work in the home with the ones closest to us.

Mother Teresa said, "If you want to change the world, go home and love your family." It has been such a blessing to have the charge to come home and love our family. Our family is stronger because of Tori's struggles. The ability to understand Tori's brain and help her gave us a chance to enjoy the gift of our daughter in new ways.

We've been receiving the care and attention of the Family Hope Center for Tori for twelve years now. Support, care, direction, partnership, wisdom, knowledge, and the drive to learn more every time is a trademark of the Family Hope Center and Matthew and Carol's team.

—*Tina Demoss, Tori's mom*

NEURO-PARENTING POINTS

- Building a support team that supplements and sustains your efforts to help your child toward growth and development is important and necessary.
- Your team should consist of people who know and care about you and your child and who respect your goals.
- Team members can include family, close friends, teachers, professionals, and anyone else who plays an active role in your child's care and support.
- Choose your team members wisely and assign them specific roles they can and want to fulfill.
- Communicate with your team members clearly and regularly so that they can meet the goals you set, complete the tasks you assign, and always keep the lines of communication open between you and among the other team members.
- Assess your team and each team member on a quarterly basis and adjust when necessary. This encompasses adding or reduc-

ing the number of team members or replacing members who
are not a good fit.

- If professionals are selected as part of your team or to serve
  your child in general, ensure that their approach to wellness and
  principles of healing align with yours.
- Parent support groups can be a great source of comfort and
  information, particularly if you feel isolated or want to be among
  others who share the challenges you face.
- If your child is attending or planning to attend school, take time
  to ensure that the school is equipped to provide appropriate
  support for your child and is open to collaborating with you to
  make the environment and experience proactive and positive.
- If necessary, consider retaining the services of financial, administrative, and legal advocates and professionals who can
  assist with government, educational, and financial benefits and
  support that may be available for your child, as well as any legal
  matters that may need consideration.

CONCLUSION

Breathe.

Often, we have to remember to breathe, and we think of ourselves as pretty normal. We think of every parent of a hurt child or adult as normal. We all want to succeed, experience growth, help our loved ones. At the same time, we don't want to leave the child, our families, or ourselves behind.

This book was many years in the making. The concepts, principles, and pathways we have laid out for you really do work.

Understanding your role as a father and mother, heading into each day proactively, and delivering a neurological approach with wisdom, with love, with humor, and with your eyes wide open leads to a happy, productive family.

Knowing you're on the correct path turns grief into hope, fear into peace, and despair into joy. Joy is when you know you know and are content to finish each day the best you can. There's a phrase some people use that we love: "Win the day."

With that phrase in mind, we'd like to leave you with our tips and recommendations for winning your own day.

- Brain injury is in the brain.
- Symptoms don't define the child.
- Labels are not scientific.
- The principles of neuroplasticity are for everyone at any age.
- The brain grows from the bottom up.
- The brain grows by stimulation and opportunity.

- Stimulating one level of the brain with enough frequency, intensity, and duration will foster the next level of brain function.
- The person who is being healed must trust the healer.
- Focus on abilities, not disabilities.
- Function determines structure.
- Nutrition!
- Physiology versus pathology.
- Execute—be consistent in your effort. If love would have solved the issue, the child would be done already. Love needs an action plan.
- Be patient with yourself and the process. With your kindness, love, patience, wisdom, perseverance, and a neuro-directed inside-out, bottom-up approach, your child can change for the better.
- Measure first using the chart—it will help you know where to begin, when to change, and reassure you when you've made progress.
- Get fit and stay fit—everyone wins when you get fit in your spirit, mind, and body. When we change, our kids can change.
- It is said that one plow horse yoked by a master can pull up to four tons, and two plow horses can pull up to twenty-three tons. Be twenty-three tons. Stay together and trust that your family has all the gifts to help each other—this circumstance will refine the gifts everyone has.
- Finally, remember this could be your proudest achievement ever.

It has been our honor and pleasure to share this journey with you. We hope this book has helped, and will continue to help you and your family in countless ways.

ACKNOWLEDGMENTS

First and foremost, Carol and I acknowledge the grace of God to finally find the time to put nearly forty years of experience down on paper. We thank our parents and siblings for their belief in us, and the great encouragement they have given us over these many years. We thank our children, who were in this together with us firsthand. We thank the many families for their love and dedication to their children.

You taught us many lessons.

We would like to thank our entire team at the Family Hope Center who continue to amaze us with their love for and dedication to healing families with us. We so appreciate you all.

And for those who have gone before us and through their work have taught us: Temple Fay, Glenn Doman, Gretchen Kerr, Elaine Lee, Master Wu, Ed Tronick, Barry Gillespie, Steven Gutstein, and the many amazing, dedicated clinicians, who have intersected our lives.

Thank you for your passion.

We would also like to thank June Clark for her support in writing the book—she was very helpful. Peter Rubie, for his help in putting this book into the capable hands of BenBella. Finally, we are very thankful for the professional team at BenBella for believing in the importance of this information and guiding us to its publication.

ABOUT THE NEWELLS

Throughout their careers, the Newells have dedicated their hearts and souls to their work and the children and families they serve. Single-minded in purpose and intent, they have brought together a team of like-minded doctors and professionals to create the Family Hope Center. The Newells observed firsthand and clinically how the brain can change and grow organically. By devising customized plans and guiding parents on implementing plan techniques, children once classified as "lost causes" have made substantial growth without the intervention of or dependence on medication.

The Newells remain committed not only to helping these special children and their families, but also toward the loftier goal of integrating neurodevelopment into schools and educational programs that serve children with special needs and brain injuries.

ABOUT THE FAMILY HOPE CENTER

The Family Hope Center is an international organization dedicated to working with (and for) parents of children with special needs and neurological difficulties. Using an evidence-based, scientific approach, the Family Hope Center educates and helps parents promote functional improvement in their children in the areas of physiological health, physical structure, sensorimotor abilities, behavior, cognition, and communication.

By combining the expertise of clinicians and therapists from multiple fields, the Family Hope Center works one-on-one with parents to create an interdisciplinary, complementary, and individualized set of guidelines to address the multifaceted challenges faced by children with developmental disabilities.

The Family Hope Center works with families to:

- View their child as a whole person, not a collection of symptoms and disabilities
- Assess the root cause of your child's developmental challenges
- Design a scientifically based program to develop their child's brain
- Put parents back in control of their child's development

Since its inception in 2002, the center has helped more than ten thousand families create better futures for their children. Across all categories and diagnoses, the clinical gains made by the Family Hope Center children far exceed national averages—even when they entered programs at a more advanced age or with a higher initial impairment than the national average.

Based in suburban Philadelphia, the Family Hope Center operates conferences and programs at their headquarters as well as around the globe, reaching parents in thirty-five countries. Due to their effectiveness and demand by parents, these programs are now subsidized or promoted by the national healthcare systems of Denmark and Norway, and expanding into Colombia and South Africa.

For more information about the Family Hope Center, visit
www.familyhopecenter.com.

INDEX